IF YOU DON'T HAVE AN ALLERGY NOW—CHANCES ARE SOMEDAY YOU WILL!

Allergies can develop at any time during your life. You may even be allergic—and suffering needlessly—without knowing it. Skin eruptions, headaches, asthma, digestive problems, arthritis, respiratory disorders—all can be caused by allergic reactions, and all can be treated and cured!

Includes diets and recipes specially formulated for allergy sufferers!

Allergies

WHAT THEY ARE AND WHAT TO DO ABOUT THEM

Jack A. Rudolph, M.D. / Burton M. Rudolph, M.D.

A JOVE BOOK

ALLERGIES: WHAT THEY ARE AND WHAT TO DO ABOUT THEM

A Jove Book / published by arrangement with
the authors

PRINTING HISTORY
Five previous paperback printings
Jove edition / October 1977
Third printing / July 1983

ISBN: 0-515-07107-2

Jove books are published by The Berkley Publishing Group,
200 Madison Avenue, New York, N.Y. 10016.
The words "A JOVE BOOK" and the "J" with sunburst
are trademarks belonging to Jove Publications, Inc.
PRINTED IN THE UNITED STATES OF AMERICA

Acknowledgments

ALL CASES related or referred to in this volume are authentic. With a single exception, they have all been drawn from our personal files. For obvious reasons, however, we have not used the real names of persons and places.

Acknowledgments must be made, however, to the many serious investigators who have spent their lives unraveling the story of allergy. To the American Academy of Allergy and the American College of Allergists, the two national allergy societies which have presented much information on allergy in forums and in journals. To the Allergy Foundation of America, now well organized and seriously disseminating knowledge of allergy to the public. To our many friends, the teachers and investigators of allergy today with whom we have exchanged views often and from whom we have learned much.

The Authors
J. A. R.
B. M. R.

Foreword

"Allergy" is a medical term denoting increased or excessive sensitivity to certain substances, such as ragweed pollen or poison ivy; to sudden changes in emotional response, or to such external conditions as excessive cold or excessive heat. These stimuli are harmless to the majority of people. Such increased sensitivity has also been noted to feathers, strawberries, cheese, eggs, perfume and soap in some individuals. Some people are born with such increased sensitivity and others have it thrust upon them. At some time in life, almost any person has an allergy, and probably 15 to 20 percent of the population will show allergic responses to several substances at some time.

While such conditions have existed for centuries, medical studies of means of prevention or treatment have been perfected to a great degree only since the turn of the century. Studies of the environment have led to improvements in air pollution and water pollution which have been helpful in certain cases. Perhaps the best example of such improvements has been in smoke abatement.

Laboratory methods have been perfected to measure the changes in various tissues by proper tests on the blood, urine, saliva and sweat. Such investigations have led to development of extracts which may be applied to the skin to produce characteristic, readily visible changes as a result of exposure to the material responsible for the allergic reaction. Other laboratory measurements have been developed to indicate the possibility of respiratory difficulties recognized as bronchial asthma, hayfever, and bronchiectasis. Almost any part of the body may be affected in an allergic state, including the skin, lungs, eyes, head and nervous system.

What is being done about allergies? *First,* experts in the field of medicine identified as "allergists" have received intensive and extensive education in learning to properly apply test procedures and to interpret such findings to determine the causative factors for allergy in an individual. *Second,* by worldwide experience and continued research publications, allergists are constantly improving their methods of identification of troublemakers. *Third,* careful studies by research workers have shown that some drugs are helpful; and certain foods or drugs are harmful to the patient. From these studies come advice regarding diets, as well as effective drugs to be used under medical supervision. *Fourth,* with continued clinical experience, it is possible to confirm the safety and effectiveness of foods and drugs in these allergic individuals, so that products may be bought over the counter to help control allergic reactions. *Fifth,* humans vary greatly; "One man's meat may well be another man's poison." This calls for astute medical study and observation of causes, prevention and treatment of allergies. Conditions which are helpful in one patient may make another patient much worse.

Based on a wealth of experience over several decades, in the treatment of thousands of patients with all types of allergic developments, Dr. Jack A. Rudolph is eminently qualified to speak to patients, their parents and their children; to explain the reasons for development of their allergic manifestations; the reasons for following certain paths of treatment; the methods of selecting the proper drugs for each patient; and the interpretation of changes in these patients during the course of treatment. Therefore, he has spelled out a useful and interesting handbook for potential as well as actual patients with allergies.

JAMES C. MUNCH, PH.D., F.A.C.A.

Contents

PART III

Introduction

IT HAS BEEN estimated that over 100 million Americans are afflicted with some form of allergic disease. Of these, approximately 20 million suffer with allergies severe enough to require serious attention. The allergy may be seasonal hay fever, asthma, eczema, contact dermatitis and other skin eruptions, digestive disturbances, arthritis or respiratory disorders. Many individuals are not treated properly, because their condition is not recognized as being an allergy.

Recent studies have revealed that such illnesses as rheumatic fever, rheumatoid arthritis, scleroderma, dermatomyositis, certain forms of nephritis, anemias and blood and blood vessel diseases resemble hypersensitivity reactions which have been produced in the laboratory. Other diseases involving the glands of internal secretion, particularly the thyroid gland, have now been shown to be allergic in origin.

Allergic reactions to drugs, especially to penicillin, are becoming quite commonplace. The increase in allergy to occupational substances has become a real hazard, both from the standpoint of inhalation and from that of contact. These conditions are preventable if serious attention is given to the factor of allergy.

The allergies have been neglected because the teaching of allergy is inadequate in most medical schools. The graduates of these schools are deficient in their understanding of allergic diseases and, therefore, fail to recognize and treat them properly. Despite the need for qualified physicians in this specialty, most medical men remain disinterested and loath to enter into the study of allergy as a life work.

Hospitals offering proper facilities for both inpatient and outpatient care are few in number. Allergic individuals require many more treatments than the average nonallergic person. There are but few scattered rehabilitation programs across the country for the allergic child and adult alike. The emotional component is often of prime importance in resolving the allergic problem, yet the assistance of psychiatrists is often difficult to obtain.

The National Institute of Allergy and Infectious Disease, a government-sponsored agency, is largely responsible for the impetus and gains in the field of basic and applied research in allergy. There is great need of more scientists to go into the research of allergic fundamentals.

This volume is written with the hope that it is meeting the challenge and assuming some of the responsibility of informing and educating the public about allergy. It is, in our judgement, supplementing the great effort being made in this direction by the Allergy Foundation of America, a national voluntary health agency established largely through the efforts of the two national allergy societies, the American Academy of Allergy and the American College of Allergists.

The phenomena of allergy and the many allergies constitute a challenge to the physician at this time. Your interest in thoroughly informing yourself as to what the allergies are, and what you can do about them, will enable you to find joy in living and to tell others of your newfound health and happiness.

PART

ONE

CHAPTER

1 *The Allergies and Case Work-ups*

WORLD WAR I had ended, and now the energies of the people were caught up in the maelstrom of fast flivvers and speculation. And then, from Tennessee, came an interruption to the cadenza of the Twenties, and, for a brief respite, the attention of the nation focused on a debate argued by two men of brilliant minds—one a lawyer, the other a minister. Central to the debate was the question: What is man?

Stirring the country, this debate was carried into millions of homes where pros and cons were argued further. But, unfortunately, there was never a clear decision. The subject was doomed to oblivion simply because it was affected by "point of view."

On the one hand, there was a man highly regarded by the ministry and, on the other, a man equally respected by the legal profession. Whereas one argued from a spiritual standpoint, the other was more concerned with the physical or tangible.

In your own mind, you will probably decide that one factor is as important as the other, and your deduction is correct. The majority of us, however, have been inclined to favor the physical point of view, for surviving on spiritual food alone is practically like living on love. It is all right until you get hungry.

Everything is proper in its place. A fine attorney may save a client's life in a courtroom, but, given an operating room, a scalpel and a harem of nurses, he couldn't remove an appendix to save the same person's life. Or a bottle of cascara may do wonders for a constipated body, although it would decline to open a stuffed carburetor.

These are not absurdities. There are uninformed individuals who do things that are equally unreasonable.

There are, for example, all kinds of motor oils. To the average person, they all look alike. Perhaps we cannot afford oil that sells for 25 or 35 cents a quart. Ah, what's this? A grocery store with a special on motor oil at 12 cents a quart. That's just fine! We pour gallons of 12-cent oil into the motor, and the car apparently starts, runs and stops the same as it ever did.

Everything is fine until one day the car won't start at all. A garage man (at $3.50 per hour) tells us that a gummy tarlike substance has been accumulating in the valves and that new piston rings are needed. He suggests that the condition may be the result of using oil made with a paraffin base.

Man as a physical being is a machine, too, and his reactions are very much like those of a machine. The similarity ceases when we realize that there is a tremendous difference between what can happen to a motor that has been fed improper oil and to a man who has been given improper food to eat and improper air to breathe.

So far as the motor is concerned, there are three alternatives: you may stop using the car, in which event the condition grows neither better nor worse; you may continue to use the car, but, sooner or later, you would have to stop; or you may call in that repairman to remove and replace the faulty parts, in which case the motor will very likely function again.

Let us see how the same alternatives apply to the human body. Mr. Smith may be very fond of sweet corn, but there is something about his internal chemistry that abhors this food. Smith has noticed the effect of corn on his body. As a matter of fact, he had seriously considered promoting it as a palatable substitute for castor oil.

Smith is an average man, and does not realize that there are other reactions to his favorite delicacy. The fact that his body throws off sweet corn ought to indicate to him that it is not wanted, but his weakness for corn supersedes his consideration for his own health. He continues to pour the roasting ears into his internal mechanism until one day something goes wrong. What is he to do? Can he stop using his body? Hardly. Can he continue to take his particular poison? Not if he becomes seriously ill.

Unlike the car owner, Smith has but one alternative. He goes to see his doctor who, like the repairman, must give him an overhauling. He will turn out almost as good as ever, but there is one reaction he will have that a motor can never experience—a psychological alteration.

His illness will undoubtedly change Smith's personality to a certain degree. He will remember how he felt. And he will have the power to observe, to report and to change.

What is this "mystic" power that common, ordinary sweet corn has over Mr. Smith? What is it that makes one man's food another man's poison?

These questions baffled the medical profession for decades. Some men believed that there was a logical answer, whereas others chose to accept such conditions as necessary evils.

The men with foresight stuck to their guns and began to prove that the word immunity could apply to garlic as well as to smallpox. It was with a great sense of achievement that they came to associate ragweed with hay fever.

As a normal outgrowth of thousands of experiments and years of research, came a new branch of medical practice, one that concerned itself with unusual reactions of the human body.

The pages to follow will present the incredible, the pathetic, the humorous, but ever significant, stories of everyday people with allergies. The interesting and unusual incidents of their lives could happen to almost everyone.

As an introduction, let us first present the true story of Dick W.

From the outset, he was an unlucky child—not from the standpoint of wealth or wisdom, but from that of health.

It was hardly 24 hours after the physician had slapped the infant's breathing mechanism into action. The nurse had just returned him to his crib after his first feeding. An hour later, a slight rash developed about the infant's scalp. The physician recognized it immediately as cradle cap—a visible indication that the child was sensitive to cow's milk. The diet had to be changed at once.

Having taken the baby home from the hospital a few days later, the proud father hastily contacted the physician to inquire as to the cause of "sniffles," especially since precautions had been taken to prevent the child from catching cold. After several questions and several replies, the doctor assured daddy that the "sniffles" were merely an inheritance from parents afflicted with hay fever.

The father did not wish to take any chances, so he

wrapped the baby in an extra, 100 per cent wool blanket. Soon the baby developed a 10 per cent annoying rash due to his sensitivity toward wool. Result—nocturnal perambulating for daddy.

A few months later, the physician was called in to diagnose an asthmatic condition in the infant. Tests showed that the baby was now sensitive to fish and nuts, although he had not eaten these foods. Mother and father exchanged glances, then looked dubiously at the doctor. It didn't seem to make sense until the physician explained that junior's contact with these two items came indirectly through the breast milk his mother had given him. She had been eating these two foods, and indirectly he had too.

A year or so passed, and the child's diet had been broadened to include many other foods. Immediately after the introduction of tomato juice into his diet, a nasty case of eczema occurred. Realizing that this condition had not existed until the child drank tomato juice, the doctor easily found the trouble.

The boy was soon old enough to play on the floor. Hardly a day had passed before the mother noticed that he was sneezing regularly. It was sufficiently warm in the apartment, and all precautions had been taken to shut out drafts. The physician, looking for other sources of difficulty, found that the cattle hair contained in the padding beneath the rug produced a reaction upon the boy's body.

Believing that the child needed a companion, the mother one day came home with a cute little Chow puppy, which remained in the household just long enough for the doctor to advise that a sensitivity to dog hair had been causing the child's asthmatic condition.

The following year, when junior was a bit older, his mother permitted him to play in the back yard. That

practice soon had to be discontinued because his inherited sensitivity toward the grass pollens had caused
an outburst of "rose fever."

A number of difficult years passed. The boy, now in
public school, took a liking to the gymnasium. After
spending many hours there tumbling on the soft, large
(but, unfortunately, dusty) mats, he found himself
annoyed with fits of sneezing and of being extremely
short of breath, both conditions resulting from dust.

Having finished high school, the boy, now a young
man, enrolled in a local college. Dad would gladly
have footed all the bills, but he couldn't afford it. The
next best thing for the young man was a night job,
and, because bakeries operate through the night, that
was just the thing. A brief, energetic search, and soon
he was working nights in the mixing room of a local
bakery.

All went well until the first time he attempted to
mix dough himself. Hardly fifteen minutes after the
first contact with wheat flour, his hands swelled to
three times their normal size. The doctor across the
street immediately diagnosed the difficulty as a sensitivity toward wheat.

Looking for another night job, the young man remembered that the morning newspaper was printed
at night. Why not a job at the newspaper plant? The
pressroom foreman was impressed with the lad's am-
bitious program, and gave him a job cleaning the
presses after the last edition came out.

This was fine. It lasted nearly a week, and then the
young man's face broke out in the worst case of dermatitis ever witnessed by the family doctor. A checkup
indicated that printing ink was the offending irritant.

Fortunately for this young man, he had been aided
in overcoming all his allergies because of the co-

operation of his parents. They realized that a better way was available to control Dick's recurring allergies. A specialist discovered the allergies and treated Dick for them.

In the following pages, the allergies will be discussed in sufficient detail to provide more complete understanding. Examples of allergens which cause some of these allergies will be cited. They represent just a few of the many on record. They have been selected for their diversity of nature, as well as for their universality of application. But first, let us trace briefly the history and background of allergies.

CHAPTER

2 *History of Allergy*

THE STORY of the allergies probably began in antiquity, but the first record of an apparent allergy was noted in the year 3000 B.C., when the Emperor of China, Shen Nung, ordered pregnant women to refrain from eating fish, chicken and horsemeat. Ulceration of the skin was thought to be due to eating these foods. Hieroglyphics on Egyptian tablets record the death of King Menes in 2641 B.C. from the sting of a hornet. The well-known adage, "one man's meat is another man's poison," was stated by Lucretius in the first century B.C. Migraine was described by Aretaeus in 110 A.D. and by Galen in 139-200 A.D. The latter described certain individuals who always sneezed in the presence of certain plants and flowers.

There is much in the biblical literature of the Old Testament which suggests dietary restrictions were observed in many cases because of the allergies they produced in the digestive system. Hippocrates, in his writings, discussed "asthma," and also stated that "it is a bad thing to give milk to persons having headache."

Many years elapsed before the effects of plants, flowers, trees, grasses, weeds and foods were noted as causing sneezing attacks and asthmatic paroxysms. In the seventeenth and eighteenth centuries, it was observed that cold could cause attacks of asthma, hives and fainting.

Early in the nineteenth century, Dr. John Bostock, a London physician described his symptoms, which were those typical of hay fever. Later, Dr. Blackley identified the cause as due to grass pollen, and did so by means of a skin test.

Early in the twentieth century, much investigation was being carried out in the laboratories in the United States, France and Germany bearing on the allergic reaction. It was found independently by most of these researchers that, when an animal is given a first injection of a foreign substance, nothing would happen; yet, giving this substance a second time, after a lapse of a few days, could produce a fatal result. The term for this serious reaction was called *anaphylaxis,* meaning without protection, in contrast to the term *prophylaxis,* meaning with protection.

Clemens Von Pirquet and Bela Schick, in 1906, made further observations of the same nature and chose the term *allergy* rather than anaphylaxis, the word allergy meaning altered reactivity, a changed state of the animal organism regardless of the cause.

Progress in the allergies was rapid after this basic understanding, and soon patients were not only being skin-tested with many substances, but were also treated successfully for their allergies.

Food allergies and skin allergies were now recognized and studied and treated after successful discovery of the causes. It has now been accepted as factual that allergy may be a potential cause of any medical condition. Although much is now known about the symptoms of the allergies and what causes them, there remains a great deal to be learned about the allergic reaction within the cells of the body, and about the action of many chemical substances which are known to participate in the reaction. Some of these are histamine, serotonin, acetylcholine, heparin and slow-reacting substances, just to name a few. Our good results in the future may depend on special drugs which will neutralize, destroy or prevent the formation of these chemicals in the body.

CHAPTER
3 How One Develops Allergy

IT HAS long been known that asthma, hay fever and migraine tend to run in families. One member may have asthma, whereas another will have migraine. There appears to be an inherited predisposition to develop an allergy. When both a father and mother have allergies, there is a probability that a child from such a union has a 75 per cent chance to develop an allergy before he is 10 years of age. When one parent has allergy, the child has a 50 per cent chance of developing an allergy before he is 20 years of age. The more remote the family history, the later in life the allergy will develop. Although the allergic tendency generally follows the Mendelian law as a dominant characteristic, there are generations that miss having allergy.

The best evidence strongly suggests that we inherit the tendency to become allergic to a foreign substance, that the nature of the substance or its source is not inherited. What one will become allergic to depends in a large measure on the degree of exposure. Many of us living in the United States may become allergic to ragweed pollen and have hay fever or asthma. In England, grasses are a more frequent offender. This is due to the higher concentration of pollen in the atmosphere.

Most authorities on allergy agree with the findings and conclusions reached, which state that the greater the inheritance of a family history of allergy the more likely will be the development of allergy in the offspring. It is also an accepted fact that one receives the predisposition to allergy and not the specific allergic disease. Descendants of a parent suffering from hay fever, may develop asthma or eczema and not hay fever.

It has been believed by a few investigators that the gene does not play a role in the production of allergy, because they have found that the frequent occurrence of the hypersensitive state, in the lower animals and in man, makes it difficult to disassociate acquired and genetic factors in its occurrence. However, recent studies in which the genes were carefully analyzed have noted that effects especially when certain drugs have been administered, are altered because of the arrangement of the genes. Therefore the adverse side effects of inherited gentic systems are now better understood. We are therefore coming to a more unified understanding of the part the genes or heredity play in allergy.

Occupational allergies demonstrate the importance exposure plays. For example, bakers may become sensitive to rye or wheat flour, laboratory workers to rabbit or guinea pig hair, fertilizer manufacturers to tobacco, DDT and castor bean dust. As the story is written, many causes of allergy will be described, in addition to factors predisposing to the development of allergy.

The kind of symptoms one develops frequently depends on the physical type of person one is, on the quantity, quality and character of the allergic substances to which one is exposed and on how they enter the body. Although heredity may play a part in the physical development, a constitutional predisposition may also exist, such as in epilepsy, diabetes or cancer. The allergies, as we have already mentioned, also tend to run in families.

Symptoms depend also on the way allergens enter the body. Dusts, pollens, animal dandruff and hairs, molds

and other inhaled substances usually produce symptoms such as sneezing, running and blockage of the
nose. They may also cause irritation and twitching of
the eyes, with itching, tearing and redness. This group
of symptoms is known as hay fever. Coughing, wheezing and shortness of breath may result, varying in
intensity from mild to severe asthma or allergic bronchitis. Continuous contact may also cause allergic skin
conditions on the face, neck and hands. Cosmetics,
furs, leather and dyes are the more frequent causes of
skin allergies. Foods will cause digestive disturbances
of an allergic nature, but will also cause hives and
migraine headaches. On the other hand, foods are also
responsible for many allergies of the nose, bronchial
tubes and the skin, reaching these areas by way of the
blood stream. Certain bodily changes take place after
infections at times, and enable the body to react more
readily to allergic substances. For example, after
whooping cough, measles or pneumonia in children,
asthma frequently occurs. When there is an infection
of the gastrointestinal tract coupled with diarrhea, un-
digested food proteins may be more easily absorbed,
causing allergy.

Certain foods cause these symptoms more often than
others. Seafoods and strawberries, for example, produce
hives more often than other allergies. Chocolate causes
migraine and other allergic headaches frequently. It
is also known that some foods, such as eggs and spices,
may be eaten on occasion and no allergy will occur,
but, if eaten often, they produce marked allergy. It is,
therefore, clear that quality as well as quantity may be
a factor in producing symptoms. Changing foods by
heat may alter both factors and change allergenicity.
When milk is boiled and given to a milk-sensitive baby,
it may then be tolerated. This is the reason for the

successes of hypoallergic milks or condensed milk in some milk-sensitive infants.

What part does the nervous system play in this discussion? For many years, doctors considered asthma and mucous colitis as disturbances of the nervous system. It has been shown that allergic persons have an extremely irritable or unstable autonomic nervous system. One part of our total nervous system is the voluntary nervous system, and is controlled by our will power. The other part is the autonomic nervous system, or the involuntary nervous system, which cannot be controlled directly by our will power. This is most important as there are also two parts to the autonomic nervous system: (a) the parasympathetic, or vagus, nerve system, which, when stimulated, can cause contraction of the eye muscles and stimulation of the glands and muscles of the bronchial tubes, stomach, small and large intestines or colon; and (b) the sympathetic nervous system, which, when stimulated, relaxes these muscles and decreases the gland secretions. In normal health, there is a balance between these two systems, so that the muscles are neither too tense nor too relaxed. When this situation is present in an allergic person, he is said to be in a "balanced allergic state."

Because the allergic individual is inclined to have a very excitable parasympathetic, or vagus, nervous system, he has been called a vagotonic individual. The nervous system of the asthmatic individual or one with mucous colitis is easily set off or triggered by an irritation. However, contact with the usual allergic substance is not essential, because nonspecific conditions, such as changes in weather, indigestion, fatigue, irritating gases, head colds and shock, will precipitate an attack of asthma or other allergies.

4 *How Allergy Is Diagnosed*

EVERYONE IS familiar with the fact that some persons develop rashes if they eat strawberries. This is not due to anything ordinarily poisonous in the strawberry itself, but to a peculiarity in the body cells of the person who eats strawberries. Certain cells are so changed that the strawberries act like a poison when in contact with them. Such cells are known technically as sensitized; the person is said to be in the sensitized or allergic state, and is called an allergic or hypersensitive individual. It should be understood that such individuals may be quite normal and robust in every other particular. Furthermore, it should be understood that the condition is a specific one. In the instance mentioned, it is only the strawberry which causes the rash.

If, for example, a hypodermic injection of egg white is administered to a guinea pig, no harm is done to the animal and it remains perfectly healthy. But if, two weeks later, a second injection is given, the animal dies. During those 14 days, the guinea pig had apparently developed a sensitivity to egg white. Post-mortem examination reveals that death was caused by an over-distention of the lungs, with entrapment of the air in the alveoli, due, in part, to spasmodic contractions of certain muscles, and, in part, to an outpouring of mucus. The guinea pig is said to have died from anaphylactic shock.

The similarity between the symptoms shown by the

guinea pig prior to death from anaphylactic shock and symptoms exhibited by persons suffering from asthma was first pointed out in 1910. It is now generally agreed that asthma, hay fever and a number of other human allergic diseases somewhat resemble anaphylactic phenomena in animals.

How Symptons Are Produced

One of the most striking facts about the history of allergic patients is the occurrence of allergic symptoms in other members of the family. Most observers report such a history in over one-half of the cases. Some believe that the tendency to allergy is inherited. This, however, has never been definitely established. Possibly, the ease with which a patient can acquire sensitiveness may be an inherited quality.

In our own series, 50 per cent of the patients had a family history of allergy. The actual proportion, however, may have been higher, because most persons recall only cases of hay fever and asthma, usually forgetting or failing to report eczema, hives or other allergic conditions in the medical history of the family. In view of these findings, we believe that most patients with allergic symptoms have a natural tendency to allergy— the sensitive state that comes about when the patient's body develops the ability to react. A person may be in the allergic state for many years before sysmptoms are manifested. Not until that patient comes in contact with an adequate dose of the specific substance to which he is sensitive do symptoms occur. Just as in the guinea pig, the shock is produced only by the particular substance to which he is sensitive. The severity of the symptoms depends upon the size of the dose, the degree of absorption and the sensitivity of the patient. The particular symptoms depend upon the organs or tissues of the body which are sensitive. If the skin is the sensitive tissue, eczema or some other skin disease will be produced; if the lung, asthma, spasmodic croup or spasmodic bronchitis; if the nasal mucous membrane, hay fever; if some portion of the alimentary tract is the sensitive tissue, digestive disturbances will result.

Many individuals possess a threshold of tolerance for the specific substance to which they are sensitive. They will not show any reaction to a small dose, developing under those circumstances what Vaughan called the "balanced allergic state." Any small additional dose may then bring on symptoms. There are also certain patients in a balanced allergic state who will develop symptoms from additional irritations of a general character.

Specific substances which can produce allergy are technically called allergens. They may enter the body in four ways: through the mouth or nose during breathing, through the digestive tract, through the skin by injection or absorption and (in the case of bacteria) by infection. Under modern conditions of life, we come into daily contact with countless substances, many of which are allergens. The air we breath always contains floating particles of many kinds, such as pollen, dust from leaves, particles from the dandruff and hair of animals, dusts produced in industrial processes and so forth. Any of these may affect an allergic patient through the mouth, nose or skin. Any food may be an allergen for a particular patient. The most common foods are the most frequent offenders in this respect. Bacteria may act as allergens.

In addition, there are many stimuli which produce symptoms when the patient is in the balanced allergic state. However, these influences bring on symptoms only when the patient has had a dose of the specific allergen which affects him. Among these irritations, are weather changes, exposure to heat or cold and certain nervous influences.

How Diagnosis Is Made

The diagnosis of any disease may be divided into two parts, the history and the examination. History is of extreme diagnostic importance in allergic patients. The age of the patient, the age at which symptoms began and the frequency and severity of attacks must all be ascertained. The home environment, the presence of animal stables or special factories in the neighborhood, the type of bedding and furniture used, all are significant. The history of attacks following some specific exposure and the existence of an allergic family history are of great importance. A carefully obtained history will usually enable the physician to be certain of the existence in the patient of an allergic state, and may afford some clues to the exciting causes.

The basis of all examinations is the investigation of every organ of the body by a physical examination, supplemented by studies of the blood and urine. This will disclose any intrinsic causes for the symptoms, such as nasal sinus disease, abscessed teeth, diseased tonsils, infections elsewhere in the body or chronic heart or lung disease, and may disclose other changes in the blood suggestive of allergy. Finally, special examinations are available to furnish clues as to the nature of the specific allergens.

The basis of the examination is the cutaneous or "skin" test. Years ago, it was observed that, if pollen was rubbed into the scarified skin of a hay-fever sufferer, an urticarial wheal or hive would develop at the site of the scratch, and that this reaction could be produced only by the particular pollen to which the sufferer was

sensitive. Later, it was determined that other substances to which the patients were sensitive would give
similar reactions, and this method is now in general
use for the purpose of affording clues to the specific
allergens in any case. When these clues have been obtained, we plan experiments in which contact with
the suspected allergen is avoided. If the symptoms are
brought under control, it is then necessary to expose
the patient to the specific allergen to see if the symptoms can be reproduced. This must be done with each
allergen which gives a positive skin test before it can be
included in or excluded from the list of specific causes.
It is in this part of the study that the cooperation of
the patient is so vital, as the avoidance of specific allergens can be accomplished only with his help.

Other Allergic Conditions

In addition to hay fever and asthma, certain other
manifestations of allergy are produced when organs
other than those of the respiratory tract are the sites
of the shock reaction.

The most common of the nonrespiratory allergies are
eczema and urticaria. Some cases of mucous colitis,
many of the so-called "gastrointestinal upsets" of children and certain joint affections are allergic in nature.
Although these conditions may exist alone, they are
usually associated with some other form of allergy.
Many asthmatics—20 to 40 per cent according to different observers—give histories of eczema during infancy or childhood, and frequently hay-fever sufferers
report attacks of hives at various seasons of the year.
Many infants with eczema are troubled by "gastrointestinal upsets," occasionally complicated by convulsions of an allergic nature.

Foods are usually the responsible factors, but other

allergens are sometimes to blame. As in other forms of allergy, the history and the skin reactions provide clues which are to be followed, as described in detail in the preceding pages. If this fails to produce complete relief, the patient should be placed on a diet containing no more than two or three foods, preferably those seldom eaten, for a period of from seven to 10 days. If the symptoms disappear, one new food is added every week, as long as no symptoms recur, until a pleasant and adequate diet has been establishhed.

Complete study of all infants and children with allergy is imperative, as, by this means, allergens which may cause symptoms later in life may be discovered and eliminated to prevent the precipitation of attacks in adolescence or adult life.

Cooperation Between Patient and Physician

The most common impediment to success in the treatment of allergic conditions is the attitude of the patient. This attitude is one of skepticism, indifference and unwillingness to cooperate fully for an extended time. We know of few illnesses in which patients, as a class, are so difficult to manage. Sufferers from tuberculosis, heart disease, diabetes or even cancer will usually go to any length to cooperate with the doctor if the essentials of treatment are explained to them. This is not often true, however, of patients with chronic allergic symptoms. This is not a specific result of the disease, allergy, but is due rather to the fact that the sickness is a prolonged one, rarely terminating fatally, that it is subject to frequent changes for better or for worse without apparent cause and that a bewildering array of drugs and "cures" is being constantly and persistently pressed upon the patient.

Few disorders can become as chronic as allergy. It

can be present from infancy through old age. Few diseases are subject to such rapid and apparently unexplainable change. Finally, few disorders expose the public to greater exploitation.

Many patients are willing to try any number of "treatments," usually remedies recommended to them highly by their friends or neighbors as positive cures. They experience so many disappointments that they eventually become unwilling to make any serious effort which requires time, sacrifice or conscientious obedience to orders. This is unfortunate for few diseases require more care, study and time, both for diagnosis and treatment, than do allergic conditions.

Unhappily, this attitude of hopelessness is not limited to patients. Many phyisicians also seem to despair of effective treatment in allergic conditions. By experience, these chronic conditions often resist treatment, only to improve spontaneously without apparent cause. The physician rightfully questions the effect of any specific therapy for a disease which often gets better without treatment. Most doctors, furthermore, have tried highly recommended remedies and have had so many disappointments that they are inclined to scoff at enthusiastic statements concerning the possibility of relief. This is unfortunate, for patients are sometimes persuaded to abandon treatment because of a casual remark made by a physician of their acquaintance.

Finally, the physician should familiarize himself with the fundamentals of allergy before undertaking the complete management of a patient; otherwise, disappointment is almost certain. Nothing could be more preposterous than the view, too widely held, that a diagnosis can be made by the use of a few skin tests, or that a cure can be effected by injecting the patient with materials which give a positive reaction. This reasoning may be correct in a very small proportion of pollen-sensitive patients, but it is decidedly incorrect when applied to the greatest number of patients, particularly those with perennial symptoms.

Methods of diagnosis and treatment which have been recommended in good faith, and which have been made as nearly foolproof as possible, are certain to fail in most cases unless they are associated with a thorough study of the individual. In this, more than in any other disease, methods of diagnosis and treatment must be modified to suit the individual patient. The same technique which succeeds in one case may fail to relieve another patient apparently suffering from the same illness. In the appendix, detailed lists of allergens are given to indicate how careful the study must be in discovering the cause of the allergy. Allergies and examples of them are presented which will allow for a greater understanding of the problem involved.

CHAPTER

5 *Special Tests to Detect Allergens*

THERE ARE several different types of skin tests, and all depend on abrading the skin slightly by pricking or making small scratches. A small amount of the allergen or suspected substance in liquid form is placed on these small abrasions in the skin and rubbed in gently. This technique is known as the prick or scratch test. When the liquid is injected between the layers of the skin, it is known as the intradermal test. The skin tests are usually performed on the arm, forearm or back of the individual. These tests are usually without discomfort and leave no scars if properly performed. If one is sensitive to an allergen, the area will turn red, swell slightly, itch and form a small hive.

In infants and children who are nervous or frightened, or in adults who have extensive skin allergies or, in general, when the skin is highly sensitive, the passive transfer test is done. A small quantity of blood is withdrawn from the allergic person. The serum is removed from the blood and prepared for sterility by proper filtration. Very small quantities of serum are then injected into a normal nonallergic person's skin in a number of areas. These skin areas will become allergic for a short time. They are marked with ink so that the location of this area is known. These areas can be tested to the different allergens and give quite accurate reactions; this is a valuable test for those patients who cannot be tested directly.

What does the skin test mean and how important is it? Although skin tests are not infallible, they are very significant when added to the other diagnostic aids used in making a final evaluation of the allergic condition. They are most valuable when a person's symptoms are due to airborne allergens such as pollens, dusts, animal danders and molds. Food reactions, though less significant, must be carefully worked out in relation to dietary habits.

Skin test reactions may indicate past, present or even future sensitivities. Lack of reaction on the skin may still not rule out a substance as the cause of allergy. The skin test is merely one aid which is of value when positive. Scratch or prick tests are not quite as sensitive as the intradermal or passive transfer tests, but they are less likely to produce such severe reactions on the skin. More than one allergen is usually the cause of reaction, and it may require great zeal and study to ferret out the many allergens which cause the allergy.

The mucous membrane of the eye may be used to determine the degree of sensitivity of an allergic person. Specific concentrations of an allergen are dropped in one eye and a control solution in the other eye. After several minutes redness, tearing and itching will indicate that a reaction is taking place.

Occasionally substances are blown into the nasal or bronchial passages to reproduce symptoms when skin tests are negative or questionable.

Ingestion of specific foods in capsule form unknown to the patient is on occasion done and simultaneous blood tests are done. The counting of the white blood cells may give some clue. If the drop from normal is more than 2000 cells within 15 minutes to one-half

hour, it may be significant. This is called the Leuco-
penic Index Test. There is some difference of opinion
as to the value of this test.

Patch-testing of the skin is done only for contact
dermatitis or in drug allergies with skin rashes. This
test attempts to simulate the skin rash by placing a
small amount of the suspected allergen in a nonirritating concentration upon the skin, fastened to it by
nonirritating adhesive tape partially covered with cello-
phane. The reaction may occur in several hours or may
take as long as 72 hours. When the patch is removed, a
small reproduction of the rash in the patch area represents a positive reaction. It is important to understand
this technique and use proper concentrations, as widespread reactions of the skin may result and be more
serious than the original rash. This test should be
applied only by those experienced in its use, interpretation and possible complications.

6 What Allergy Tests Mean

Convulsions and Asthma from Egg

FIVE-YEAR-OLD Allen Y. was rushed to the hospital. His sudden attack of convulsions had frightened his parents, but, within an hour, the child had responded to emergency treatment and was resting fairly well. The parents were still not satisfied. They feared a recurrence and, worst of all, they feared the cause.

The next day, the family physician examined Allen thoroughly and found him to be in excellent health. This added to the mystery, for the doctor admitted that the convulsions of the previous day had baffled him.

"You're positive that you have been watching Allen's diet," suggested the doctor. "You remember the severe asthmatic attacks he had just a year ago whenever he ate eggs."

"I'll never forget those attacks," replied the mother. "That's why I've been so careful to see that he doesn't eat anything containing eggs."

"I'd like you to think back and tell me everything Allen ate prior to his attack of convulsions," requested the doctor.

Each item of food was listed.

"You're sure there wasn't something else?"

"Oh, yes," Mrs. Y. reminded herself. "During the afternoon, when I took him marketing with me, I bought him a box of animal crackers."

"Then that makes things clearer," said the doctor. "You probably didn't realize when you bought those animal crackers that the baking powder used in making them contain egg."

Mrs. Y. was greatly surprised.

"But then, if it were the egg in the animal crackers, why didn't he just get an attack of asthma?" she asked.

"That is easy to explain. You see, during the year he stayed away from eggs, his lungs strengthened. The weakness of sensitivity toward eggs was still present. The convulsions he suffered yesterday were just a different expression of that sensitivity," replied the doctor.

Mrs. Y. smiled sheepishly. "From animal crackers," she mumbled. "It looks as though I'll have to learn more about what goes into the things we buy."

We have already mentioned that, if an injection of egg white is administered to a guinea pig, apparently no harm has been done to the animal, and it remains perfectly healthy. But, after a period of two weeks, if a second injection is given to the animal, it will die. During these two weeks, the guinea pig has developed a sensitivity or allergy to egg white. The lethal dose of this substance then causes swelling of the lungs, cutting the breathing mechanism from operation through spasmodic contraction of the muscles and an outpouring of mucus.

It was just this sort of experiment that led to the discovery of the causes of asthma and other allergies.

You may wonder why there is an allergic tendency in some individuals and not in others. For that matter, why are some people hot-tempered whereas others can remain cool under any circumstances?

There has never been established definite proof that a tendency toward allergy is inherited. Some believe it is, whereas others are not so sure. An examination of the case records of a large number of patients has shown that 50 per cent of them gave a family history of allergy. It is reasonable to suspect that a large portion of the remaining 50 per cent overlooked such symptoms as eczema, hives and other less prominent allergic conditions.

A person may be in an allergic state for many years before symptoms of his sensitivity appear. Not until he comes in contact with an adequate dose of the substance to which he is sensitive do symptoms occur. Just as in the case of the guinea pig, the killing shock is produced only by the particular sensitive substance.

The degree of severity with which one reacts to his personal poison depends upon his degree of sensitivity, the size and dose and the extent to which his body absorbs it.

The particular symptoms depend upon the organs or tissues of the body which are sensitive. Thus, as stated earlier, if the skin is the sensitive tissue, eczema or some other skin disease will be produced; if the lungs, asthma, croup or bronchitis; if the membrances of the nose, hay fever; if some portion of the alimentary canal is the sensitive tissue, the resulting disturbances will be digestive.

Select several persons at random. Make a strong statement about religion, and observe the individual reaction. The extent of each one's reaction may be considered his tolerance level. Naturally, the tolerance level of one may be far above that of another.

The same holds true in allergy. Each individual is endowed with a tolerance level. Those who are fortunate can go a long way before running into allergic difficulties. Some, to the best of their knowledge, never do. This kind of individual may not show any reaction to a small dose while he is in a balanced state of allergy, but just give him a small additional dose of the irritating substance, and he overflows his tolerance level, displaying symptoms of allergy.

These specific substances which produce allergy, or allergens as we have referred to them, may enter the body as previously stated, in one of four ways: through the mouth or nose during breathing, through the digestive system, through the skin by absorption and (in the case of bacteria) by infection.

Under modern conditions, we come in contact daily with countless substances, many of which are allergens. The air we breathe contains floating particles such as pollen, microscopic dandruff, the hair of animals, dust from leaves and dusts produced in industrial processes. All or any of these may affect the allergic person through the mouth, nose or skin. As we have shown in cases presented later in this volume, practically any food may be an allergen if it finds its way into the right person.

But there is another way in which an allergic reaction can overreach the tolerance level. Let us suppose that you are allergic to sweet corn. You may eat one ear of it without sensing a reaction. However, along comes a secondary stimulus, such as an abrupt change in temperature, or a physical change or possibly even an emotional alteration of your mind. This secondary stimulus is sufficient to reduce your tolerance level, and, the first thing you know, your allergy is in operation.

Upon numerous occasions throughout this volume we have referred to "skin tests" and "sensitivity tests." Perhaps a question has developed in your mind in regard to these terms, so we're going to clear up the matter once and for all.

What happens, you may ask, when one visits the office of an allergist?

The physician's first job is diagnosis of the case. This is done in two principal parts—history and examination.

In allergy cases, history is of extreme importance. The doctor will ask his patient: "What is your age? What is the nature of your disturbance? When did you first notice the symptoms? How often do you have the attacks? How severe are they? Are they worse at one time during the year than at other times?"

These, and many more questions concerning home, environment, presence of pet animals, proximity of certain factories and the type of furnishings in your household, help give the physician a clear picture of the situation.

As may be expected, the basis of the examination is a thorough physical checkup, supplemented by various tests. This procedure will generally disclose any intrinsic causes for the allergic symptoms, such as sinus infection, abscessed teeth, diseased tonsils, chronic heart or lung disorders or any other type of infection within the body.

Ultimately come the special tests designed to furnish clues as to the nature of the specific allergens that may be causing the trouble. These are the "cutaneous" or "skin" tests.

Devised a number of years ago, these tests are in general usage among the allergists.

Hundreds upon hundreds of food, pollen, dust and bacterial concentrates are applied individually by means of a hypodermic needle. Some doctors apply the tests to the individual's back, whereas others use the muscular upper arms for their testing ground. Either is satisfactory. At each meeting with the physician, the patient is painlessly injected with about 20 different allergens. After 10 or 15 minutes, the physician "reads" his interpretation of each injection, and evaluates it on a chart. A negative reaction is recorded with a zero. A slight reaction in the form of an irritation, rash or hive about the point of the injection may be evaluated as a "plus," "one plus," "two plus" and so on, depending upon its apparent significance.

This procedure continues until all available tests have been made and all possible clues obtained. This completed, the physician then sets up a plan of treatment for his patient. This is designed principally to exclude all contact with the suspected irritants.

After the allergic condition is brought under control, it is necessary for the doctor to learn whether he can produce the reaction himself. He does this by injecting into the patient's arm quantities of the allergens which gave positive reactions in the tests.

The doctor of allergy is not a magician, nor is the hypodermic needle a magic wand. Anyone who is sincerely interested in eradicating the causes of his periodic or perennial discomfort will find that this can be done only through teamwork. The nature of allergy is such that a victim is scarcely ever in immediate danger of his life.

Sufferers from tuberculosis, heart trouble, diabetes or cancer know that their lives are at stake, and they go to great lengths to follow the doctor's orders. The allergist doesn't usually expect the same treatment from his patients.

As we have said, the fact is that few disorders can become as chronic as allergy, for it can be present from the earliest days of infancy through old age. Few ailments are subject to such rapid and apparently inex-

plicable changes, and few lend themselves to more
public exploitation.

The individual who gets "burned" by a number of
these "remedies" eventually becomes unwilling to make
any sacrifices, or to bend a serious effort toward eradicating his difficulty. This is unfortunate because there
are few diseases that require more care, study and time,
both for diagnosis and treatment, than does allergy.

TWO

7 *Bronchial Asthma*

Asthma from Rye Flour

FRED M. was out of a job again. This was the third job he had lost within a month. This in itself was hardly as important as the fact that Fred was over 50 years of age and knew no other work. He had started as a baker's apprentice right after leaving high school and, since that time, all his life had been at this kind of work.

He was alert, he possessed a certain amount of ingenuity and he was well-versed in the art of baking, all of which had assured him of steady work throughout the years. He liked his work, and the fact that he had remained at one job for 27 years was, in itself, sufficient testimonial.

But, suddenly, striking as a bolt of lightning from behind the clouds, he was called in to see his boss. "Fred," began the employer slowly, "I'm afraid I'll have to let you go."

For a moment Fred stood bewildered. Many thoughts raced through his mind. "I—I don't quite understand," he said.

The employer reiterated his statement. "This is your last day here. I'm giving you two weeks' pay to hold you over until you get another job."

"But—I like it here. Twenty-seven years I have worked here. I don't know any other work," Fred protested. "Where will I go? What will I do?"

"I'm sure you'll get another job right away, Fred," assured the other man. "Perhaps another bakery. There are several other big ones, you know."

Fred felt that there was something more to this than appeared on the surface, but, out of respect for his employer, he accepted the facts as they were and, after choking out a brief farewell, turned and left the office.

As Fred trudged toward the door of the bakery, he made up his mind that he wasn't through. His reputation as a baker was known by all the tradesmen. His recipe for rye bread was the envy of all the other bakeries in town.

Convinced that he had not lost his usefulness, he marched straight to the next largest bakery in town, where he was promptly employed.

This gave Fred a certain sense of satisfaction and self-reliability, and once more he felt happy. But this was not to last long, for hardly two weeks had passed when his dismissal was again requested.

A third and fourth bakery retained the man for similar periods of time, but nobody would give him a reason for his failure to hold a job.

Just before leaving his last place of employment, he accidentally overheard two of his recent co-workers discussing him.

"Damn shame about Fred," one of them said. "Swell guy."

"Got canned because of his cough, they tell me," commented the other.

"Yeah. Guess the boss couldn't take a chance. Maybe he's got T.B. or something. Gotta be careful."

Fred was shocked. He had never thought his cough was anthing serious. Right then and there he decided that this was not the end for him. Had the employers only told him that this was the reason for his dismissal, he could have explained. They were not to blame. They only tried to avoid hurting him, he figured.

His general health was good, and this prompted him to believe that his cough was not really serious. Yet he had to do something about the situation. He had not been able to save, and the thought of charity was repugnant.

The thing foremost in his mind was the affliction that had cost him his job. His first visit to a doctor's office convinced him of one thing. The physician assured him that he did not have a lung ailment, but that was the extent of the diagnosis. Believing that Fred was suffering from the effects of a bodily irritant, the doctor referred him to a specialist.

In a short time, the new physician learned by means of tests that Fred was highly sensitive to the thing he had handled most while he worked in the bakery—rye flour. The mere contact of this flour with the delicate membranes of his nose and throat caused him to choke and cough. His lungs had been the fuse box of his body; consequently, a rash had developed there due to his constant association with this particular food.

Fred listened with interest to the doctor's diagnosis.

"Do you think you can convince my former employer that I am not seriously ill? Perhaps he would take me back."

"If I thought it would do any good, I'd be happy to do so," replied the doctor. "As a matter of fact, I don't believe he could really be convinced, and, if he were, the job would do you more harm than good."

Fred looked disappointed. "What am I to do? I haven't the money to live on."

"I'm going to handle your case," replied the doctor. "I believe that the State Industrial Commission will pay compensation on a case of this sort."

For several years, the Industrial Commission had been confronted by just such cases, but it had never been thoroughly convinced that these cases came under its jurisdiction. By furnishing sufficient medical facts, the physician proved that Fred's illness and his loss of employment had originated industrially.

Other individuals employed in industry, who, at one time or other, have developed bodily reactions against the things they work with, have benefited from this precedent.

Bronchial asthma is a frequent allergy which occurs seasonally and also the year around. It is, on occasion, associated with other allergic conditions. True allergic asthmatic attacks result from exposure to allergens either by inhalation, ingestion, injection or by absorption of bacteria from a focus of infection. There are conditions arising from heart disease, obstruction of the bronchial tubes from within or without, which resemble allergic asthma, and, from which, true asthma must be differentiated if correct treatment is to be undertaken.

True asthma results from spasm of the bronchial muscles, swelling of the lining or mucous membrane and thickening mucus within the bronchial tubes. This produces the shortness of breath, the prolonged phase of breathing out and the wheezing or musical sounds while breathing.

At the outset, the acute attack is manifested by tightness in the chest, with cough and shortness of breath. Thickened phlegm of a gelatinous type is often present. When it is brought up, the patient feels better. This result occurs when the attack subsides or appropriate medication is given. The attack may occur suddenly, day or night, often without warning, following exposure to an allergen, or subsequent to whooping cough, pneumonia, measles, the common cold or sinus infection.

The examination may reveal nothing abnormal in the early stage of asthma between attacks. During an attack, the individual will be sitting up and leaning forward, pale, cold and sweating and extremely breathless. The neck veins appear prominent. In long-standing cases, when complications have set in and emphysema is present, the chest is shaped like a barrel. The chest on percussion or tapping has a hyper-resonant sound. Wheezing is often heard without a stethoscope. With a stethoscope, all types of musical and noisy sounds are heard. There are special crystals known as Charcot-Leyden crystals or Curschmann's spirals in the sputum. There is also an excess of a special white blood cell, the eosinophile, in the blood stream.

The allergens are recognized from the history and special skin tests. The physical examination, food idiosyncrasies and seasonal, environmental, temperature and weather changes should be evaluated. In addition, possible emotional factors, nasal infection, foci of infection and endocrine imbalance should be carefully investigated, as they may precipitate an attack.

In some patients the attacks develop gradually, beginning with symptoms of a "cold in the head," progressing gradually into the lungs. Many of these are mistaken for attacks of bronchitis, especially in children, in whom the attacks may be for years so mild as to mask the asthmatic nature of the condition. However, usually in these cases, one notices wheezing breath sounds which are seldom found in simple bronchitis and the presence of which usually indicates asthma.

Some patients have asthma only at certain seasons of the year, as, for example, a complication of hay fever or pollen asthma without hay fever, occurring during the latter part of August. Others may have attacks at any season of the year. Patients presenting attacks at the same time every year suffer from "seasonal" asthma; those who may develop symptoms at any time or who have continual attacks are said to have "perennial asthma." The perennial asthmatic may suffer most severely at some one season—a characteristic of perennial asthma with the seasonal exacerbations.

In order to develop asthma, one must have (a) the allergic state and (b) contact with the specific exciting cause to which the patient is sensitive in quantities sufficient to produce either immediate allergic shock or the balanced allergic state.

The physician must determine all of the exciting causes which may enter the body from the outside (extrinsic causes), and all of the abnormal conditions in the body which may tend to disturb the allergic balance (intrinsic causes). Asthma may be divided etiologically into three groups: extrinsic, intrinsic and combined. Purely extrinsic cases are those in which there are no physical deformities or defects in the body, and in which the exciting causes enter from the outside through the air or food.

Extrinsic cases are the least difficult to diagnose and treat. These patients show seasonal variations often depending on changes of residence from one house to another, or from one community to another. A complete set of skin tests usually affords many clues to the specific exciting causes. When this information is obtained, the life of the patient is rearranged in order to exclude the exciting factors from the environment. The patient is then brought into contact with the suspected materials one at a time to see if attacks can be reproduced. If, under these circumstances, an attack occurs, it is necessary to avoid the reacting substance indefinitely in order to keep the patient free of asthma. If, in spite of all efforts to remove the suspected influences from the patient's environment, attacks continue, it is obvious that removal has not been complete, or that other active allergens are present.

To determine the completeness of removal of the known allergens, the household furnishings and the wearing apparel, frequent sources of allergens, are investigated. To do this properly, the physician must have a thorough knowledge of the materials used in the manufacture of both usual and unusual clothes and furniture. Goat hair, horsehair, feathers, silk, fur, wool and cotton are present in almost every home in some form or other.

Most of the furs found in homes are derived from the common furbearing animals, which have been altered by plucking and dyeing to resemble the more expensive and rarer kinds, under which names they are often sold. Some of the furs commonly altered and sold under names of superior furs are:

Natural	*Altered and Sold as*
Hare, dyed	Sable or Fox
Hare, white	Fox
Rabbit, white	Ermine
Rabbit, white, dyed	Chinchilla
Rabbit, sheared and dyed	Sable / French Seal / Electric Seal
Muskrat, dyed	Seal, Electric Seal / Hudson Seal
Muskrat, pulled and dyed	Mink, Sable
Mink, dyed	Sable
Marmot	Mink, Sable, Skunk
Opossum	Beaver

To determine the presence of other and unknown allergens, samples of dust are collected from various parts of the house; these samples are extracted and skin tests are made with the extracts. The dusts are collected in the following manner.

The cloth bag is removed from a vacuum cleaner. The machine is then operated for a minute or two to free the working mechanism of any dust which may be present. A piece of muslin is tied on in place of the cloth bag, and the machine is operated directly or by means of attachments, so as to collect a tablespoonful of dust from the mattress, pillows and linen of the patient's bed. The muslin is then removed, folded and labeled, and another clean piece is tied on in its place. A sample is obtained in a similar way from the living room rug, from the bedroom rug, from the automobile and from such other sources as might suggest themselves after a survey of the surroundings. Dust is often collected also from the working environment.

If any of these dusts give positive reactions in the patient, and negative reactions in normal individuals, the source of the dust is eliminated from the environment, and a survey is made once more to determine the effect of this change.

Sometimes, this method fails and it is then necessary to move the patient to a specially prepared room in a hospital, where the air is so free of all particles that the patient cannot possibly receive any harmful substances through the air. By means of special filters, similar conditions may be produced at home. The patient remains in the special environment until it has been determined with certainty whether inhalant factors are responsible for attacks. During all this time, the diet should be arranged in accordance with the clues derived from the history and the skin tests.

When the conditions necessary for the control of the attacks have been determined, these conditions should be maintained indefinitely. Efforts to raise the tolerance to specific allergens, although temporarily successful, are never lasting, and are of chief value when it is impossible or impractical to free the environment of the offending material.

The treatment of purely intrinsic asthma consists of the surgical eradication of all removable areas of infection, and of attempts to improve the body health by hygienic measures such as regularity in living, attention to excretory functions, simple nutritious diet and ample fresh air and exercise. In these cases, the aim is to assist temporarily in the raising of the body's tolerance.

The combined form is relatively common. It consists of a combination of the extrinsic and intrinsic types, in which the extrinsic causes are usually the more significant, as in most instances the intrinsic causes are insufficient to produce symptoms until the body has been placed in the unbalanced allergic state by contact with doses of the specific exciting causes. Treatment consists of a combination of the methods described for the extrinsic and intrinsic types.

Heart Failure and Asthma

For nearly two years, Harry B. was under medical care for severe asthma. He had become almost a complete invalid, unable to do more than walk a few steps before his breath gave completely out. Upon the insistence of his wife, who had learned of a similar case "cured" by an allergist, her physician referred this man for study and care.

There was no question about the allergic history in Harry's case, for he had had hay fever and an asthmatic

cough for most of his 48 years. He had a sister with
asthma and his father had hay fever. His allergy tests
and blood tests certainly confirmed the fact of Harry's
strong allergic condition—but that was not the whole
story.

When he was 10 years old, Harry had spent five weeks
in bed with a rather prolonged illness. He had a continuous fever, nose bleeds, sore throat, enlarged glands
and painful swollen joints. The family physician said
he had an enlarged heart with a loud murmur. The
condition was thought to be rheumatic fever.

For a number of years, Harry seemed to be short of
breath on exertion of even the mildest degree. He could
never play with the kids, and he was nicknamed
"wheezy."

It was difficult, but, upon examination, it was ascertained that his allergy alone could not account for the
type of heart murmur he exhibited, nor could it account
for all of his shortness of breath, cough and wheezing.
With more refined techniques, X-rays of the interior of
the heart revealed that the mitral valve of the left side
of the heart was nearly completely obliterated, preventing normal circulation. It was further determined that
all of the factors were right for Harry to undergo heart
surgery in which the mitral valve would be "cracked"
(as the surgeons call splitting and enlarging the opening). Harry made a dramatic recovery and his circulation was restored to nearly normal. His allergy is still
being treated and controlled to keep all strain off the
heart. Harry walks 25 blocks to and from work now
without distress.

This case illustrates the existence of two distinct conditions, rheumatic heart disease and allergic asthma.
Harry could have lived with his allergy without treatment, but he could not have lived without the

recognition of his serious heart disease. Harry has certainly had 25 years added to his life.

Asthma from Peppermint

An exceptionally interesting case was that of John K., an important business executive in a large midwestern city. His family physician referred him to an asthma specialist only after months of unsuccessfully attempting to locate the source of his difficulty.

One of the first things Mr. K. said to his new physician was, "I hope you can find the trouble with little or no loss of time. I'm a busy man. I can't afford to waste time, and the only reason I'm here is that my asthmatic attacks make it difficult for me to work."

The physician convinced Mr. K. that he was not a magician, and that he could only accept the case if he had absolute cooperation. John K. agreed under protest and proceeded to give the facts concerning his ailment.

"When do you get your attacks?" asked the doctor.

"Generally twice a day," was the reply.

"Last long?"

"The first one is fairly brief. It comes between nine and ten in the morning, and lasts for about 45 minutes. The afternoon attacks are more provoking. They generally last all afternoon."

"Are there any days when you have no attacks?" the physician asked.

John K., reflected momentarily. "Sometimes I manage to get through an entire Sunday without having much trouble. That's probably because I spend most of the day sleeping."

"Is there any other time when you are not bothered by these attacks?"

"Yes. When I'm away on business trips, I find that the attacks come less often," replied the patient.

"Haven't you ever tried to figure out why?" the doctor asked.

"I've been too busy to think about it," John K. replied with an embarrassed chuckle.

"It seems to me that a thing which affects your health and, incidentally, your business activity would merit more consideration," suggested the physician.

"You know how it is, Doctor. Most of us take our health for granted," Mr. K. replied.

"When you are away on business trips, do you alter your living routine a great deal?" queried the doctor.

"Not at all," said John reassuringly, "I make it a point to stick as closely as possible to my regular routine."

"Yet your attacks come less frequently while you are away?"

"It does seem strange, but it's true."

After extracting considerably more history from the patient, the doctor proceeded with the routine task of making skin tests for the various foods. Nothing significant appeared in these tests.

A day-by-day record of the asthmatic attacks was given to the physician regularly. Oddly enough, the morning attacks occurred invariably between the hours of nine and ten, and the afternoon attacks usually began between one and three o'clock.

Here, at least, was something for the doctor to work with. He set himself to the task of learning precisely what Mr. K. did within the hour preceding each attack.

Very often the obvious goes unnoticed, and here was an excellent example. Several weeks passed, and John K.'s asthmatic attacks continued with their customary regularity.

The doctor traced every avenue of possibility. He even spent several days at Mr. K.'s home, watching him closely from the moment he arose in the morning until he left for the office. But all was in vain. One day the physician decided to go along to the office with John K., believing that a new clue might present itself. It was a tedious and apparently hopeless task sitting in the patient's private office all morning, making note of every move he made, and everything he handled. It was doubly tedious because of the fact that John K. was a very busy man, and had practically no time to converse with the physician.

The morning had passed, and along with it the morning asthma. Noon arrived.

The doctor noted the time. "If you'll pardon my intrusion, Mr. K.," he began, "isn't it about time for lunch?"

Mr. K. smiled. "Lunch? That's something I have no time for." With this, he slid open his desk drawer and removed a small, round package.

"This is my lunch," explained John K. with a chuckle, indicating the small package.

The doctor learned that these were dextrose wafers.

"Not the best way to eat lunch," apologized Mr. K., "but, when you're busy, a few pieces of dextrose candy go a long way toward replenishing your energy."

The doctor agreed, but at the same time wondered whether this was the clue he had been waiting for. He reflected that the patient hadn't eaten any of those wafers in the morning, and, furthermore, that there was nothing in pure dextrose that might have such an effect.

He returned the candy to Mr. K., who promptly opened the end of the package, offered it to the doctor and took one himself.

The candy was good, thought the doctor as he chewed it. Suddenly an idea came to him.

"Of course!" he exclaimed. "Why didn't I see it before?"

"See what?" said John K.

"It was so obvious that I overlooked it. Mr. K., what flavor is this candy?"

"Why—peppermint. Helps the digestion they say."

"It's also a spice," reminded the doctor, "and some people can't eat peppermint, just as others can't eat black pepper."

John K. reflected for a moment. "But I only eat these at noon. How would that account for the morning attacks?"

"Your toothpaste—what flavor is it?"

"Holy smoke!" said John K. slowly. "Peppermint."

"And you eat these dextrose wafers every day except Sunday?"

"Right."

"And on Sundays you don't have more than one attack," explained the doctor. "That attack is from toothpaste."

John K. sat silently in amazement for several moments.

It was a mere matter of routine detail to check the doctor's diagnosis. An extract of peppermint injected into the patient's arm confirmed the fact.

Needless to say, John K. no longer suffers from asthmatic attacks for he carefully avoids peppermint-flavored foods.

Food Allergens

The food allergens encountered in our practice are listed in the Appendix not for the purpose of alarming the reader, but rather to open his eyes and mind to facts.

Each of these foods has the potentiality of altering one's health to the point at which a physical or mental breakdown is inevitable.

If this list makes you aware of the fact that even the most trivial quantities of the most common foodstuffs become poison when reacting with certain human bodies, then it serves its purpose.

One person cannot eat English walnuts without losing his wind. An infant sensitive to cow's milk is no longer troubled with bodily rashes when changed to goat's milk. The gum-chewing stenographer who punctuates her typing with 30-second sneezing finds that, by eliminating chicle from her diet, she is no longer afflicted with this reflex. The sweet-toothed housewife, who intends to surprise hubby with a nice, rich devil's food cake and samples about half of it herself, often finds that the chocolate flavoring has been the cause of gastric disturbances. And the corpulent gentleman with a lust for starch foods learns that potatoes, not business worries, have been bringing on those dizzy spells by indirectly affecting the semicircular canals in his ears.

Some persons have tongues which resemble the topography of a relief map because of the elevations and depressions caused by some particular food allergen.

The greater number of food sensitivities occur in mild and apparently harmless, but annoying forms. Headaches are common, yet they signify that something is not functioning properly. When they occur with regularity, it is time to investigate the underlying cause. The same can be said for any other apparently minor ailment, for it is the constant weakening of one part of the body that evokes serious complications.

Asthma from Feathers

A woman and her two young boys entered the office.
"I'd like to see the doctor, please," she announced
to the receptionist.

The girl at the desk smiled. "Do you have an appointment?" she asked.

"No. I was sent here by another doctor. I'd like to
see him about my two boys," replied the woman curtly.

"What is your name, please?" asked the girl.

"Mrs. T.," was the brief reply.

In a moment, the girl was in and out of the physician's private office. "The doctor can see you now,"
she said, gesturing toward the open doorway.

In the private office, the woman seated herself opposite the physician, while the two boys proceeded to
familiarize themselves with various objects about the
room.

"I was sent here by Dr. R.," began the woman. "He's
a nerve specialist, you know."

The doctor assured her that he knew this.

"It's about the boys that I came to see you," she
resumed. "But I'll tell you this—I still think it's a nerve
specialist I need for them."

"Let's start at the beginning," suggested the physician. "You may be correct, but I'll be better able to
tell when I know all the facts."

"Well, they both have nervous stomachs," the woman began.

"Are they subject to particularly rigid discipline at
home?" asked the doctor.

"No. They get their own way most of the time.
They're pretty good boys for that age. They're eight
and ten. Of course, they aren't angels, you understand,
but then what boys are at that age?"

"Just how does this nervous stomach come about?" asked the doctor.

"That's what I want to know," the mother replied. "All I know is that they both wake up coughing in the middle of the night. At first I thought they had colds, but I soon found out that I was wrong. Then, they complained that their stomachs were jumping up and down."

"How long has this been going on?"

"Nearly a year," answered the woman. "I first took them to Dr. L., a nerve specialist but, when he wasn't able to help them, he called in Dr. R. for a consultation."

"Many physicians refer their patients to us when they come up against stone walls," said the doctor. "I don't say this egotistically; I say it so that you might realize how many ailments are due to specific bodily sensitivity."

"I can't think of anything the boys might be sensitive to, but, if you believe there is a chance of discovering something of that nature, I'm willing to have you try," offered the woman.

The boys were energetic and somewhat difficult to work with. They could ask more questions in five minutes than a dozen quiz programs. These details were all recorded by the physician, for they convinced him that a certain amount of nervous energy was being burned constantly, and he knew that individuals of this type were generally subject to the development of sensitivities.

The ordeal of running the regular food tests was finally completed after several weeks, and the boys were fortunate. There wasn't a thing that had to be eliminated from their diet.

The contact tests were a bit easier since the boys

were already accustomed to the procedure, although they still asked a lot of questions. Again there were no indications of sensitivity, so the bacterial tests were made. The results were the same.

By now, the mother was growing more and more skeptical.

"It does look as though we have hit a stone wall again," she offered.

"I don't give up that easily," the doctor replied. At the same time, he observed the two youngsters through the open doorway to the reception room. They had begun to amuse themselves by playing catch with one of the soft pillow seats of a reception room chair.

As the physician meditated on the next avenue of examination, he noted that the smaller boy, having been hit in the face by the pillow, began to sneeze.

"I'm going to make a strange request," the doctor began.

"If it's something to do with curing the boys, all you have to do is name it," replied the mother.

"I'm coming to your home tonight; I have a theory that I want to check before making my further tests."

Since this was agreeable, the woman and her children left the office.

That night, after the boys were supposed to be asleep, the doctor stood by their door. For a time, all was still. Then he heard soft sounds of restlessness within the boys' room. Several words were mumbled, then there was a muffled giggle and, presently, the doctor heard strange sounds, as of a rug being beaten.

After several minutes of this, the doctor took the boys by surprise. He came into the room and switched on the lights. The parents followed in time to see the boys battering each other with their pillows. The boys were as sheepish as a couple of puppies caught doing something they knew was forbidden.

Turning to the parents, the physician laughed. "This is one time I'd rather you didn't scold them," he said. "They solved their problem for us."

"What effect would a pillow fight have on their stomachs?" asked the father.

"Sensitivity toward the stuffing in those pillows. From the odor in the air, I'd say they were pine-filled," replied the doctor. "The reaction could have appeared anywhere, but their point of least resistance is their stomachs. If you'll bring the boys to my office tomorrow, I shall verify what I've told you."

"But how can they be cured?" asked the mother anxiously.

"The treatment? That depends upon the degree of cooperation we can get from the boys. There will be two steps. We must have their faithful promise that there will be no more pillow fights, and at the same time, we must cover their pillows with a dust-proof casing."

A suitable degree of cooperation between the physician and his patients over a period of several months brought fruitful results. The nocturnal coughing eventually disappeared, and so did the "jumping stomachs."

CHAPTER
8 *Hay Fever*

GEORGE K. was warned never to call at our office again when summer came. He was an extremely allergic person suffering from severe asthma. Sensitive to grasses and ragweed pollens during each of two previous summers, he was advised to take hyposensitization treatment so that he would be free of this difficulty. Even though hay fever and asthma put him out of action for the entire summer, George was stubborn, and, after he managed to survive his sickness, promptly forgot his experience.

At eight o'clock in the evening on a Fourth of July, with the road slightly wet from a moderate rain, George's wife telephoned. "George is dead," she shouted. She was hysterical and wanted us to come at once. It would normally take about 25 minutes to drive to George's house in good weather, when the streets were dry, and not on a holiday with heavy traffic. But we were lucky, and the traffic, lights and lanes all appeared to open up. We reached his home in less than 25 minutes. (Why such a rush when George was supposed to be dead?)

He looked dead to all intents and purposes. Relatives were present and last rites had been given by a clergyman. He was blue, turning white; he was not breathing; he had no palpable pulse; no heart sounds could be heard.

The training and intuition of a physician keep one trying. We promptly gave George a large injection of adrenalin directly into his heart muscle, then caffeine sodium benzoate and more adrenalin. It seemed like an eternity, but heart beat and pulse started to return, imperceptibly at first, but in a gradually stronger way. Color and breathing began to return.

This very dramatic incident made George a most faithful patient. We have often wondered whether the doctors have fully recovered.

Hay fever is the name given to the symptoms produced by contact of pollen with the allergic, upper respiratory mucous membrane. A more scientific name is pollen disease. It affects about one per cent of the population, and is characterized by attacks of sneezing, watering and itching of the eyes, discharge of watery secretion from the nose and itching of the nose, throat and the roof of the mouth. Hay fever is usually seasonal in nature, recurring annually, beginning and ending about the same time each year. When it is very severe, it may be accompanied by asthma, and may even exist in the form of asthma without nasal or ocular symptoms. This so-called pollen asthma is a rare condition.

Pollen was proved to be the cause of hay fever by Dr. Blackley in 1873. Fortunately, for most of us, only a few pollinating plants satisfy the requirements necessary for the pollen to be significant in the production of hay fever. First, the pollen must contain a precipitating factor in hay fever. Second, the pollen must be windborne. Third, the pollen must be produced in large amounts. Fourth, it must be light in order to be blown large distances. Fifth, it must be a widely distributed pollinating plant. Ragweed is, by far, the greatest offender in this regard.

There are three principal hay-fever seasons in the United States, corresponding to the pollination of three plant groups, trees, grasses and weeds. In some parts of the United States, the tree-pollinating season begins as early as January and, in some, as late as April. It may last two to three months. The early summer or grass-pollinating season begins as early as March or as late as June, and lasts approximately two months. The fall or weed-pollinating season begins as early as June or as late as August, and lasts two or three months. These seasons depend on location. In the Southeast, for example, there may be two grass-pollinating seasons.

Decorative and other flowers, such as the rose, sunflower, chrysanthemum and dahlia, are frequently thought to cause hay fever. Beautiful flowers are insect-pollinated, the pollen being heavy and scant. Close contact may cause an aggravation of symptoms, but, otherwise, it is not a serious factor in the cause of hay fever.

The same special care and thoroughness must be carried out in discovering the cause of hay fever as in asthma. Careful history and a physical examination, with special attention to the eyes, nose, sinuses, throat and lungs, urinalysis, blood count and chest X ray, are musts. Many years ago, we discovered that only 30 out of 100 patients are allergic to one pollen alone; the other 70 patients have other allergens as causes of the hay fever. This explains the many failures in hay fever treatment, whether by the conventional or the more recent "one shot" treatment.

The history of characteristic attacks recurring annually at the same season is sufficient for diagnosis. Although the symptoms of hay fever are nasal, there need be no organic abnormality; and examination be-tween attacks usually shows an entirely normal nose.

Having determined that a patient has hay fever, the physician must find out to what pollens he is sensitive and to which of them he is sufficiently exposed to ac-count for the production of symptoms. To do this in-telligently, one must be familiar with the flora of the territory, must know the hay fever-producing plants, their pollinating seasons, the relative amounts of pol-len produced by each and their symptomologic im-portance.

Pollen is the male element in the fertilization of plant seeds. All plants may be divided into two groups with respect to their methods of pollination: (a) those pol-linated by insects, and (b) those pollinated by the wind. The insect-pollinated plants have inviting flow-ers and sticky pollen. Because of their odor, color and sweetness, they attract insects which carry pollen on their feet and wings, and fertilization from the male to the female portions of the flowers occurs. These plants produce only small amounts of pollen, and, under natural conditions, their pollen is not found in the air, so that these flowers, in general, do not cause hay fever except when they are cut and used for decorative pur-poses in homes. Under these conditions, pollens may be scattered as the flowers dry. Treatment here is simply a matter of eliminating such flowers from the home.

The wind-pollinated plants have inconspicuous flowers. Their pollen grains are light in weight and are produced in great abundance. They depend on gravity and the wind for the proper distribution of the pol-len, and, as nature is solicitous for the survival of all plants, she produces excess pollen which the air con-tains in large amounts during the warm months. The plants most likely to cause hay fever are very abundant pollen-producers, and their pollen is light enough to be carried long distances by the wind. It has been estimated that a fifteen-mile-an-hour breeze will blow ragweed pollen five miles; and this pollen has been found in the air at a height of 10,000 feet.

Three groups of plants are the chief causes of hay fever: trees, grasses and weeds. Trees pollinate in the early spring, and are likely to cause symptoms of about two weeks' duration between February and April. The grasses bloom from late April to early July, and cause symptoms during that time. The weeds cause symptoms from mid-August until the first killing frost.

Certain trees, grasses and weeds are found exclusively in certain restricted parts of the country. These may cause symptoms at times other than those specified below.

Spring hay fever: A few warm days in March or April are likely to usher in the pollination of trees. Persons sensitive to some of these pollens will begin to have symptoms. These symptoms are usually mild, and, as the season is short, little treatment is required as a rule. To find the cause, it is necessary to know what trees are found in the patient's environment, which ones are pollinating at the time, and to which pollen the patient is sensitive.

Summer hay fever: About five per cent of all hay-fever patients have the summer type, often erroneously spoken of as "rose cold." This condition begins during the last week of May or the first week of June, at the time when the early roses are in bloom. Observing the beautiful rose, we blame it for the symptoms, but this ignores the inconspicuous bloom of the grass which is the real cause. Patients who are sensitive to one grass are likely to be sensitive to all members of the grass family, of which there are several hundred. For this reason, it is imperative that the physician know the names and pollinating seasons of the grasses indigenous to the territory in which the patient lives.

In Cleveland, Ohio, for example, there are four major grasses. The earlier symptoms are due to the pollens of June grass and orchard grass, and the later ones to those of timothy and red top. Sweet vernal grass, which is common in New England, and Bermuda grass, which is common in the South, do not grow in northern and central Ohio and are unimportant as causes, although almost all patients will give positive skin tests to their pollens.

Fall hay fever: Fall hay fever begins in the northern areas about August 15 and is the type from which 90 per cent of patients suffer. It is caused by pollen of plants of the Compoitae group, the chief representatives of which are giant and short ragweed. Cocklebur is also an occasional offender. Goldenrod, sunflower, and other decorative plants which are members of the group do not cause hay fever, although they are frequently suspected. The symptoms, which begin about the middle of August, tend to become more and more severe until they reach their height about Labor Day. This peak lasts for a week or two, and then gradually declines until the first hard frost stops further pollination, thus terminating the symptoms. The more pollen in the air, and the more one is exposed to it, the more severe the symptoms. Patients vary considerably in their sensitivity to pollen. For the same exposure, the symptoms will be mild when tolerance is high and severe when tolerance is low.

There are three methods of treating hay fever: (a) by the removal of the patient to an environment which is free or relatively free of the pollen to which he is sensitive, (b) by raising the tolerance to a level which will allow freedom from symptoms in spite of the inhalation of pollen and (c) by a combination of these two methods.

The first method has been in use for many years. It is customary for those who can afford it to go away each year during their season of symptoms to one of the "hay-fever resorts." These are places in which there is little windborne pollen of the hay-fever plants, either because these plants do not grow there, or because all grasses and weeds for a number of miles surrounding the resort have been cut to prevent pollination. They are usually primitive places, providing little more than the absolute necessities for living—so that they are seldom places where one would choose to spend a vacation. However, hay fever causes so much distress that suffers are willing to tolerate inconveniences in order to be symptom-free.

There are certain disadvantages about "hay-fever resorts." As more and more people go to them, and as the surrounding territory becomes increasingly occupied, land is cultivated and weeds grow in the wake of cultivated plants. Some grass and weed pollens then appear in the air and the resort loses its value for any except mild sufferers. The severely ill must then move on to resorts in still more primeval areas. At most "hay-fever resorts," for example, only about one-half of the hay-fever sufferers are completely relieved, because there is sufficient ragweed pollen in the air to produce symptoms in patients whose tolerance is low.

Because of the expense and inconvenience of making a long journey, many persons have tried to set up "hay-fever resorts" at home. One of the methods is to confine the patient to a room in which all doors and windows have been tightly closed in order to reduce the amount of pollen by excluding fresh air. Another method is to transfer the patient to a downtown hotel, where the airborne pollen concentration is less than it is in the residential parts of the city. The first method is unsatisfactory because few persons are willing to forego fresh air for an indefinite period of time to secure only partial relief. Removal to a downtown hotel affords inadequate relief and is as expensive as a trip to a "hay-fever resort."

Recently, some air filters have been made available which, without interfering with ventilation, effectively remove all of the pollen from the air coming into the room. The patient installs a filter in his bedroom and starts it in operation a few days before the usual onset date of his symptoms. He then sleeps in this room, going about his ordinary business affairs during the daytime. As the season advances and more pollen apears in the air, he will find it necessary to remain for increasing lengths of time in his bedroom. For the very sensitive patient, as many as 22 hours per day may be necessary to afford relief at the peak of the season. Some persons find it convenient to have both their homes and their offices equipped with filters so that they remain in filtered air from 20 to 22 hours a day. Those using this method should curtail their outside activities during the entire hay-fever season; they should avoid automobile and train trips, should not play golf or tennis and should remain in filtered air as much as possible. The principle of this method is to keep the daily dose of pollen below the patient's tolerance, so that he remains in the balanced allergic state.

The second method depends on increasing the patient's tolerance. It consists of repeated injections into the patient of increasing doses of pollen extract, in order to teach the body, as it were, to tolerate amounts equal to, or in excess of, doses which will be inhaled on any day during the hay-fever season. There are several difficulties in this method. First, the physician must know with certainty the exact pollen which is producing the patient's symptoms. Second, the pollen extracts must be potent. Third, the patient must be able to tolerate a sufficiently large amount to produce the desired results. Usually from 20 to 40 injections are required. Treatments are administered daily, every other day or every three or four days over a period of several weeks or months until the patient is able to tolerate sufficiently large doses to insure prevention of symptoms. If the final dose is too small or if the treatment is stopped too early in the season, very little relief will be obtained. The "one shot" treatment is now under careful study, and may be an improvement on the above.

Many physicians administer pollen extract injections supplied by commercial biological laboratories. These extracts are potent, and their routine use protects 25 per cent of cases. Experts, who use larger and more frequent doses, are able to protect a large majority of patients. However, the tolerance obtained by any injection method is evanescent and disappears quickly following the last injection; in some instances, it lasts no more than a week, and ordinarily persists only for from four to six weeks. These injections, therefore, must be repeated every year, as the tolerance acquired one year is likely to be lost before the next hay-fever season. It is for this reason that the year-around method of treatment is employed.

The third method is a combination of these two. Since only 25 per cent of patients receiving pollen allergen injections have their tolerance raised sufficiently to escape all symptoms, it is necessary that 75 per cent of these patients have, in addition, a few hours of filtered air daily in order to remain comfortable. For this group, fewer hours in filtered air will be necessary than for the average patient who has received no treatment directed at raising his tolerance.

Review of all three methods demonstrates again that the treatment of allergic diseases consists in so reducing the dose of the specific exciting cause, or so increasing the tolerance, as to produce in the patient the balanced allergic state.

CHAPTER

9 *Perennial Allergic Rhinitis*

MANY PEOPLE complain of "chronic sinus disease," "chronic catarrh," "frequent colds," coryza, or "post-nasal drip," and "bad breath." These may be perennial nasal allergy or "year-round hay fever." This condition may be clearly recognized as an allergy if there is constant or periodic nasal blocking, associated with a watery mucous nasal discharge and thicker postnasal drip. These signs are frequently preceded by bouts of sneezing. If the discharge becomes thick and yellow, an infection has been added to the allergy. If these conditions are neglected, a cough develops, with congestion in the chest, wheezing and shortness of breath. Often, headaches over the forehead occur and may be very painful.

The nasal obstruction is frequently the most distressing symptom of perennial allergic rhinitis, since it is frequently associated with mouth-breathing and the uncomfortable feelings of the mouth and throat caused by the excessive dryness. It is made worse often by exposure to fumes, dusts, changes in barometric pressure, temperature and humidity.

On examination, we find swollen, pale mucous linings over the interior nasal bones, with a layer of thin, watery mucus. If the condition is neglected, yellow pus is often noted, as well as small fleshy growths known as polyps. Removing the polyps alone, without caring for the underlying allergy, is useless, a sad lesson many sufferers learn after frequent nasal operations. The polyps will return unless the allergic cause is removed.

If the nasal allergy is not corrected, the sinuses often become involved. This occurs because of the swelling in the nose, with the impairment of normal function and the resulting superimposed infection. Treatment in addition to allergic management must be aimed at clearing up the infection by frequent washing of the sinuses or putting a permanent window into the sinuses. A study of the nasal secretions will help reveal the amount of allergy, or of infection present. These studies and others aimed at finding the responsible allergens and removing them when possible, or receiving injections to lessen the person's sensitivity, will, in the greatest majority, markedly improve or "cure" the individual. The patients who have been carefully studied and treated emphasize the points made in this discussion.

Sneezing from Pencil Wood Shavings

Bill H., employed in the accounting department of a large retailing firm, had no sooner seated himself at his desk when the mucous membranes of his nose became irritated. First there was one sneeze, then another and another. There must have been seven or eight in a row, and his co-workers began their customary ridiculing. Bill made no attempt to conceal his resentment.

"There must be some flowers in here," he said. "I can smell them and, besides, my nose doesn't lie."

Everyone defied him to find even one little flower in the entire office. It was the middle of December, and the people just weren't plucking flowers from any garden.

This business of sneezing had grown to nuisance

proportions, and Bill H. decided not to tolerate it any longer. He reasoned that he must have "rose fever," and he decided to find out for certain. He went to see the physician who was already treating him for hay fever and went through a series of tests, but there was nothing to indicate that flowers were causing his trouble.

Poor Bill! It was up to him to get more information for the doctor, so he returned to the office. All afternoon, he sat dejected at his desk trying to figure out what smelled like flowers that was not flowers.

Days later, Bill, toying with a lead pencil, happened to place it within smelling distance of his nose. "It's this pencil!"

"What's that?" joked someone. "Are there some flowers hidden inside the pencil?"

"Just about," replied Bill as he reached for the telephone and called the doctor. "Doctor, I think I have a clue," he said enthusiastically.

"What's that?"

"I believe it's the shavings in the pencil sharpener around the office that have been giving me trouble," he explained.

Bill presented his reasons, and agreed to bring in a box of the shavings so that the doctor could make a testing extract. Bill was right. When tested, he showed a strong reaction.

The next question was what to do? Bill couldn't just quit his job because of a few pencil shavings. Besides, he would have the same trouble in any office.

The next morning, he went in to see the manager of the accounting department, told of his experiences of sneezing, smelling flowers that weren't there, and eventually finding the cause of the reaction.

"I suppose you'll think it's crazy," Bill said. "But,

after all, it's for the good of the company to eliminate the cause of my sneezing."

"You're right," said the manager. "You would probably do better work if you didn't spend so much time sneezing, but what can we do? We can't stop using pencils."

"W-e-e-ell," began Bill hesitantly, "would you consider using mechanical ones?"

The manager sat pensively for a moment. "That isn't as foolish as it sounds, Bill. I'll have the purchasing agent look into the matter."

"But, in the meantime—" Bill paused.

"In the meantime," repeated the executive, "we'll remove the pencil sharpener next to your desk and instruct the night custodian to empty all sharpeners in the department every night so that there won't be any occasion for anyone to empty them during the day. That ought to keep pencil dust to a minimum."

"Yes, sir, it ought to," agreed Bill.

And it did. Bill's sneezing attacks came less and less often, and then, when the department inaugurated the exclusive use of mechanical pencils, Bill's troubles were practically over. Yes, his work became more efficient also.

CHAPTER
10 *Allergic Bronchitis*

THIS CONDITION cannot be diagnosed without giving very careful consideration to the conditions of the nose, throat, bronchial tubes, lungs and heart and aorta that can produce coughing in an individual. Such conditions may be eliminated by a careful history, physical examination and X rays of the chest.

Allergic bronchitis usually starts early in infancy or childhood as a cough which is persistent, without evidence of serious changes in the heart and lungs from infection or foreign bodies. The patient usually has an associated perennial allergic rhinitis, hay fever or bronchial asthmatic attacks. There may be wheezing with this cough. Bronchial asthma, emphysema or bronchiectasis frequently follow untreated allergic bronchitis.

It is a condition which, like the other respiratory allergies, may be perennial year-around or seasonal. If it is associated with infection, the condition is often called asthmatc bronchitis. Some consder this a bacterial form of allergy, whereas others consider it strictly an infectious bronchitis. If there is an associated allergy, together with a history of good general health, absence of fever, a nonproductive cough, a negative tuberculin test and essentially negative X rays, there is not much doubt of allergic bronchitis. A careful study of all other possible conditions should be made before a final diagnosis is made. The following interesting case illustrates the need for minute attention to detail.

This is the story of 10-year-old Joan M., an only

child. Joan's parents were not wealthy, but Mr. M. had a supervisory job which paid him adequately. Since Joan was the only child they could have, the parents showered her with attention. They gave her everything and guarded her health constantly.

It was with consternation and bewilderment that they suddenly found their daughter losing weight and acting generally sluggish. Joan was hurried to the family physician, who examined her thoroughly but could find no immediate cause for the sudden alteration of the child's health.

"Have you been feeding her well-regulated meals?" the doctor asked Mrs. M.

"The same as always, doctor," she replied. "You know that I have taken the best care of Joan."

The physician agreed. "Yes, but sometimes we can kill a person with kindness," he reminded her.

"Joan isn't spoiled," said Mrs. M. "We've just tried to do our best for her."

The doctor prescribed vitamin concentrates and kept the girl under constant observation for several months, but her weight continued to drop and the child developed a dry cough.

Her lungs were X-rayed, but the pictures were clear. Another thorough examination failed to indicate the source of the trouble, so the doctor began to think about a consultation with a specialist.

During the next few weeks, Joan submitted to all the standard food tests, the pollen and dust tests and the bacterial tests, but all gave negative reactions.

The physician leaned back in his chair and looked at the worried faces of Mr. and Mrs. M.

"We've done just about everything to help Joan, but we haven't hit upon the right thing," the doctor told them. "We'll have to check on her environment."

The parents couldn't quite understand what could possibly be wrong with the child's environment, but they were agreeable to anything that might help.

"All right, then," said the doctor, "let's begin with you, Mr. M. Exactly what kind of work do you do?"

"I'm plant superintendent at the B— Packing Company," he replied. "We manufacture food extracts."

"What particular extracts do you handle yourself?"

"Well, none in particular. I only get around to see that things are running right," Mr. M. answered. "Sometimes the machines break down, and I have to get them back into operation as quickly as possible."

"What kinds of machines do you have?" the doctor asked.

"Several," said Mr. M., enumerating. "There is the grinder, the pulverizer and the extractor."

The doctor interrupted. "Would you say that the pulverizer turns the food into a dust?"

"Well, yes," replied Mr. M. "It practically has to be a dust before it goes into the extractor. That is where other ingredients are added and the extract produced."

"Are the grinding and pulverizing machines covered in any way?"

"They can't be. The men are constantly adding raw materials to them."

"Does the plant have some sort of exhaust system to keep the air clean?" asked the doctor.

"Plant's too old for that," answered the man. "They have talked about an air-conditioning system, but they keep putting it off."

"What kinds of extracts do you make at the plant?"

"Oh, all kinds. You see, there are several divisions. Until eight months ago, I worked at the fruit flavor division. Then I was transferred to the vanilla extract division. That's where I am now."

"You say vanilla extract?"

"That's right."

"That's made from the vanilla bean, isn't it?"

"Yes, and it's an interesting process. You ought to come out to the plant sometime and let me show you through," suggested Mr. M.

"That's exactly what I was thinking, and the time is right now," replied the doctor.

At the plant, the doctor exposed several culture media to the air around the grinding and pulverizing machines. Back in his office an hour later, he examined the cultures under the microscope and found them to be thick with microscopic vanilla bean dust.

At Mr. M.'s home that evening, the doctor asked: "Do you change clothes before you come home from the plant every day?"

"No. My job isn't a dirty one. I always wear the same suit to work."

"I have reason to believe that Joan's trouble is being caused by the vanilla bean dust you carry home on your clothes, and there are only two ways to prove it. First we'll try a skin test, using the vanilla concentrate, and, if there is a reaction, you will have to help me prove that vanilla is Joan's personal poison."

The doctor made the test and found, as he had suspected, that Joan showed a marked reaction toward the extract. The father verified this finding by wearing a different suit for work than he did in going to and from the plant. The idea was to eliminate all traces of vanilla bean dust in the home.

Within the two months following, Joan began to pick up weight. She lost the dry cough, and gradually returned to the normal, healthy state she had enjoyed before her father was transferred to his new job.

CHAPTER

11 *Bronchiectasis*

THE MOST common symptoms of bronchiectasis are cough, profuse expectoration and hemoptysis (coughing up blood). A diagnosis of this condition is made by the symptoms, physical examination and chest X rays. However, a bronchoscopic examination with instillation of a special oil containing iodine will confirm the dilation of the bronchial tubes.

That allergy is a factor in bronchiectasis has long been recognized. The allergic management associated with good medical treatment will revert many cases to the dry stage, if the bronchi are too dilated and the condition has been present for a long time.

Thorough investigation in suspected cases of bronchiectasis is a must and should include a complete history, physical examination, X rays of the chest, bronchoscopy, complete allergic surveys and essential laboratory examinations, including the preparation of autogenous vaccines.

Management includes environmental control of the allergens, hyposensitization and injection of the autogenous vaccines, postural drainage with expectorants, possible bronchoscopic aspirations and, in some cases, surgical removal of the affected portion or segment of the lung. Climatic change may be beneficial; a warm, equable climate has been of help.

The importance of allergy must be emphasized in all cases of respiratory tract afflictions, as patients with major allergic manifestations can develop bronchiectasis. The following case presentation will illustrate this condition.

Asthma and Bronchiectasis

Jane R., at 57, had seldom known many comfortable days in her lifetime. She had had repeated chest colds with cough, wheezing and much expectoration as far back as she could rember. Because she spat up blood some 30 years before, she ended up in a T.B. sanatorium. Although the tubercle germ was never found, she spent about nine months in bed, without much improvement in the cough and expectoration. As the years passed, she continued to have repeated episodes of coughing and expectoration of multicolored phlegm and blood. This had now become associated with severe episodes of asthmatic attacks.

. The years of illness were beginning to take their toll, and repeated attacks now required hospitalization, as her difficulty in breathing could no longer be controlled at home. X rays revealed some changes in her bronchial tubes and lungs. Her family physician called in a specialist in bronchoscopy, but the consultant would not recommend the passing of the bronchoscope, for she was so ill that she apeared to be dying.

The cause of Jane's illness had to be found, and we were asked to evaluate her problem. Certainly she was too ill for skin tests at this time. Even if we found the causes of her allergy, she probably could not benefit from the treatments at such a time.

She was placed on heavy doses of cortisone and antibiotics. She was given intravenous feeding of glucose, ACTH and aminophyllin salt solution. Other medication was given to loosen and thin her mucus, and to reduce the swelling in the bronchial tubes. Jane began to improve, and was soon able to have a complete allergic study.

Treatment for the allergies was begun, and soon she was again hospitalized, but this time in good physical condition. Bronchoscopy and the injection of a special oil into the bronchial tubes was done, filling defects which were X-rayed. Bronchiectasis was found.

A careful evaluation of Jane's long history and a physical examination led us to the conclusion that her lung defects were congential (that is, that she was born with them). The associated allergy had allowed infection to occur, with the result that yellow-greenish phlegm formed. Since the condition was congenital, we believed it was limited to one lung. This opinion was concurred in by the chest surgeon, who removed two segments of the lung. The operation was followed by an uneventful recovery. This, we believe, was due to proper pre- and postoperative care, which included necessary allergic management.

Today, Jane at 57 is healthier that she can ever recall being. She now lives a normal life, except for her regular allergy injections. Incidentally, she has a totally changed, outgoing personality, and desires to help others.

12 *Allergies of the Skin*

Atopic Dermatitis

THIS IS a special type of allergic skin disease that is usually associated with asthma and hay fever. Members of the patient's family often have some type of allergy. This might be said to be like asthma or hay fever of the skin, with the same allergic causes requiring similar methods. Usually, the causes are food, inhalant, animal danders, pollens or molds. Foods are usually most significant in infancy, and, as the child reaches adulthood, the other allergens become more significant. Special tests are often required to determine the allergens.

Atopic dermatitis has been classified by some authorities into three stages: infantile atopic dermatitis or eczema; juvenile atopic dermatitis; and adult atopic dermatitis, called by some neurodermatitis.

Infantile atopic dermatitis occurs from birth until two years of age. The rash appears usually first on the face, with small itchy blisters. It quickly spreads over the entire face and neck, but the eyes and the area about the mouth remain clear of the rash. In most cases, the rash spreads to the sides of the legs, wrists, arms and buttocks. In severe cases, it may spread over the entire body. Because of the itching, there are often many scratches, oozing and crusting. This makes the infant very restless, but, as a rule, does not appear to disturb his general well-being. In many infants, the atopic dermatitis spontaneously clears up by the age of two. However, the recovery is often only temporary, and recurrences are frequent through adolescence and adult life. It is best to make an early and determined effort to find and control the allergy during infancy.

Juvenile atopic dermatitis may be a recurrence from the infantile state or may develop independently. The areas of skin involved are the face, forehead, eyelids, around the ears, neck and chest, the bends of the forearms and the backs of the knees and wrists. The rash is usually dry, scaly, thickened, pigmented and, often, wrinkled. The itching is very severe, and, as a result of scratching and irritation, the skin thickens and secondary infection often results, with scabs and a yellowish discharge resembling impetigo.

Adult atopic dermatitis is similar in many respects to the juvenile type. The difference is largely that it has been present so much longer and the rash is more chronic, with a bluish or grayish color in the areas where the skin is thickened. There is considerable dryness and generalized flaking or scaling of the skin. There is usually considerable scratching from the rubbing and itching. There are periodic intensifications in the symptoms. Occasionally, there is an increase in the skin rash in the winter. Due to marked itching at night, the patients tend to be quite nervous, although otherwise in fairly good health.

It is usually necessary to differentiate atopic dermatitis from several skin diseases which look like it, such as seborrheic dermatitis, contact dermatitis and neurodermatitis. Except for contact dermatitis these conditions are not allergic and will not be benefited by allergic treatment. Local skin care and treatment are very vital for the ultimate "cure" of the allergy. Treatment must also include any emotional factor, as well as attention to general health, dentistry, good bowel habits, avoidance of overfatigue and excessive night life.

Contact Dermatitis

The skin is constantly exposed to many harmless substances, and few are primary irritants. It requires one or more exposures to a substance to prepare the skin for subsequent contact dermatitis. This form of skin disease is probably the most common type of skin allergy. Patch-testing will, in most cases, reveal the causal allergens and their removal will result in cure.

The start of contact dermatitis is usually on the exposed surfaces of the skin. A sudden appearance of redness with extreme itching is soon followed by swelling, blisters, weeping and crust formation. If infection is added, there will be pus in the blisters. This is the acute type seen in poison ivy, oak or sumac cases. With subsidence of the acute symptoms, the condition, if not cured, will reveal scaling and redness of the skin, with thickening of the affected areas due partly to the irritation and trauma of the scratching. Later, the skin will become shiny and show bluish or purplish pigmentation.

The location of the contact dermatitis will have some effect on the type of eruption, and will also enable one to suspect the possible allergic agent causing the trouble. If the face in involved, cosmetics may be suspected. Pollens, plants, and dusts tend to affect the exposed areas like the face, neck and upper and lower limbs. Clothing containing dyes and fillers diluted with perspiration causes contact dermatitis where contact is direct. Dress dermatitis usually affects the skin

of the sides of the neck, the folds of skin under the arms
and the bends of the elbows and chest. Wearing shoes
and socks can quite logically result in contact dermatitis on the lower part of the legs, the insteps of the
feet and the toes. The backs of hands, forearms and
face are usually involved in occupational contact dermatitis. Although the condition is at first localized to
the area of contact absorption of many chemicals
through the skin, it may result in involvement of all
of the skin. Sodium dichromate, mercury, formaldehyde, quinine and many other chemicals can do this.

It is easy to recognize poison ivy dermatitis and
wrist watch band or rubber glove dermatitis. There are
others that are less obvious and require a most careful
analysis of the present and past personal history as well
as the family history of the occupational contacts and
medicines that are used frequently, such as laxatives
containing mercury, phenolphthalein, headache medicines, tonics containing iodine, sedatives, Fowler's
solution containing arsenic, cough mixtures and in-
jectable medicines, such as penicillin, vitamin B and
other drugs.

Contact dermatitis may resemble many other skin
conditions from which it must be differentiated. There
are other allergic skin diseases that require a different
type of treatment and skin diseases resembling contact
dermatitis which cannot be benefited from allergic
management.

The allergens responsible for the contact dermatitis
must be identified. Those related to seasonal occur-
rences, such as pollens and plants, are important.
Periodic remissions or exacerbations of the dermatitis
may give clues. Being away from the environment, contacting certain substances with regularity, using dyes or
paints in weekend work at home, special hobbies, such

as gardening, golfing and photography—all these offer suggestions for allergy. Contacts in the home, such as detergents, soaps, bleaches, turpentine, mineral spirits, furniture polishes, disinfectants, plants, pets, floor waxes, furniture, plastics, house dust, clothing, curtains, drapes, benzine and other cleaners, weeds and grasses, also offer problems.

Certain occupations involve substances likely to be causes of contact dermatitis. Telephones, business machines, dictaphones, carbon paper, pencils and dyes are sometimes implicated. Schoolteachers contact chemicals, chalk and inks; photographers contact developing solutions; beauticians contact cosmetics, waving solutions, dyes and hair tonics; bakers contact cereals, chemical, fruits, sugar and eggs; florists contact plants and flowers and barbers contact hair tonics, soaps, metals and sterilizing solutions. Service station attendants and mechanics contact gasoline, oil, grease, soaps, chemicals and cleaning materials. A carpenter will contact woods, glue, stains and varnishes, and a bricklayer-tile-setter will contact cement, lime, clay and dyes. Printers, lithographers and engravers will contact inks, cleaning fluids, sodium bisulfide, chromates, ammonia and other chemicals. Druggists, physicians, nurses and veterinarians will contact medicines, chemicals, rubber gloves and many other substances.

Patch tests are the means of determining the cause of the dermatitis in most cases. There are, however, precautions which must be observed in using these tests, as they can produce serious scars and dangerous extensive skin disease in inexperienced hands.

The finding and removal of the causative allergen and the clearing of the rash is the certain proof that a given agent has caused the dermatitis. In the following illustrations, cases of contact dermatitis are described.

Dermatitis from Nickel

A large, well-built man stood in the center of an inferno known as open-hearth plant No. 3 of the W— Steel Works. The white-hot flames from the furnace doors cast their scorching rays upon his sweat-soaked body, which was stripped to the waist.

The man's keen, deep-set, blue eyes shone as they focused upon a stop watch. Presently, lifting a whistle to his mouth, he blew three shrill blasts, then timed a crew of men for 60 seconds as they loosed a quantity of limestone into the bath.

Again there were three shrill blasts, and the man's work was finished for another fifteen minutes. As he left the furnace room, he brushed perspiration from his burning body.

"Look at 'em! Look at these darned sores," he said to a fellow worker. "And when I sweat, it's just like the fire in that furnace."

He had a nasty rash which practically covered the front of his body from the shoulders to the waistline, including both his arms.

"Hm, sure is an awful lookin' rash ya' got there," remarked the other man. "Doin' anything for it?"

"Doin' anything!" exclaimed the large man. "I'd be the happiest guy in the world if I only knew what I could do."

"Didja see the doctor in the front office?" asked the other.

"Yeah, he thinks it's heat rash. Says it'll go away by itself. Says to eat a lot of salty food."

"Well?" said the other man expectantly.

The afflicted man shrugged his shoulders. "I eat pretzels an' potato chips, an' more pretzels an' more potato chips, but every time I go into that furnace room, these sores come out again, and, man, what I mean, they sure burn! You know, I don't think the salt or the heat has anything to do with it."

"Aintcha got a family doctor? Maybe he c'n tell ya what ya got," suggested the fellow worker. "Sometimes these company doctors run into things that ain't exactly in their line. After all, they ain't only but human."

"We haven't got a family doctor, but my wife's been takin' the youngest girl to a doctor for hay fever. Maybe next time I'll go along. Who knows, maybe I got hay fever." He laughed.

"Naw!" replied the other man seriously. "That's with weeds. They ain't no weeds in here."

"Aw, I'm only kiddin'," apologized the large man.

So, the next time Mike D.'s wife took young Elsa for a hay-fever treatment, Mike went along. At the doctor's office, he remarked to the physician about his trouble.

"What sort of trouble?" asked the doctor.

Mike laughed. "I got hay fever of the skin."

"Wait," interrupted the doctor. "It may not be as funny as it sounds."

"You said it, Doctor!" exclaimed Mike. "Right now, it only itches, but, when I get to work at the hearth, it really burns!"

"What itches and burns?" asked the doctor.

"All around here," replied Mike, demonstratively pointing to the affected regions of his body.

The physician insisted upon examining Mike. After a lengthy questioning, he said: "The joke's on you, Mike. You have hay fever—a different kind of hay fever —and I'd like to find out what's causing it."

Mike needed little persuasion, and the physician began immediately to test for specific sensitivities. Row upon row of tests were made during the next few weeks. Not a single positive reaction resulted.

Then came the contact irritants. There was not a pollen in the world that reacted against Mike. Nor was his body averse to the numerous kinds of dust.

The long list of standard test items having been exhausted to no avail, the doctor braced himself for another of those battles with the unknown.

"Mike," he began, "I'm going to find out what causes your trouble, but we'll have to be patient."

"That's all right, Doctor," Mike replied in his good-natured manner. "Take as long as you like."

When Mike went to the plant that night, the physician accompanied him. "You see, Mike," explained the doctor, "I've got to know what things you work with at the plant. If your rash gets worse when you go to work, there is obviously something in the place that doesn't agree with you."

"Maybe it's the boss," joked Mike.

"Maybe," agreed the doctor. "We'll know soon enough."

Both men stripped to the waist before entering the open hearth plant for the late shift. As they checked into the torrid room, Mike paused long enough to introduce the doctor to the night superintendent.

"Boss, meet my private doctor. He's gonna find out what's makin' me itch all day and burn all night."

There was a cool nod from the superintendent. "You'll find it awful hot in here, Doctor," he remarked. "Stay away from the furnace. There's canned Hell inside." He handed Mike his whistle and stop watch.

Inside the furnace room, the doctor asked many questions. He learned that there were at least eight kinds of metal being used in the room. He also noted a number of other things. Several hours of this was all the doctor could stand, even with periodic rest periods. He felt that he had secured the information he wanted.

"Be at my office next Friday, Mike," he told his patient.

"Why so long?" asked Mike.

"I'll need time to prepare some extracts," explained the physician.

The doctor was sure he would soon know the source of his patient's trouble. The following five days were spent in preparing extracts of iron, vanadium, chromium, aluminum and several other metals.

The next Friday when Mike appeared at the office, he was tested with each metal, but one by one, they showed negative results after a 72-hour period.

Believing that he was on the right track, the doctor continued to make patch tests with the different metals until suddenly his face beamed. "That's it! Mike, we have it!"

"What?" asked the patient.

"The metal that's been causing your trouble."

"Gee," said Mike, "what is it?"

"Nickel," was the brief reply.

The light faded from Mike's face. "Are ya sure, Doctor?" he asked.

"Sure as you're alive," replied the doctor, indicating a large red area surrounding the point where the metal extract was placed against the man's arm.

"I don't know," said Mike skeptically.

"What don't you know?"

"Well, you see, we don't use any nickel in the plant. There ain't a thing we mix that's got nickel in it," he explained.

"There must be." said the doctor convincingly. "I'm

going with you tonight, and we're going to locate that nickel."

That night, with the assistance of the superintendent and Mike, the doctor scrutinized the plant carefullly for traces of nickel. There were none. The doctor watched Mike work. In his bewilderment, he subconsciously noticed Mike preparing to give the signal for pig iron. Whistle in his mouth, and his eyes glued to the stop watch in his hand, he stood motionless for a moment, then let out three shrill blasts.

Each blast seemed to say to the doctor: "Here—here —here," and finally it came to him. That whistle! "Mike," he called, hurrying toward the man. "Mike, when you said it might be your boss that didn't agree with you, you weren't far off."

"What do you mean?" asked Mike.

"I mean that the boss has been giving you a nickel-plated whistle and a nickel-plated stop watch to work with every time you come in here. That's where the poison is coming from."

"Well, I'll be—" was all that Mike said.

The doctor's theory was checked and found to be correct.

Mike's request for a wooden whistle and a silver-plated stop watch was quickly fulfilled, and, within a very short time, the rash disappeared completely from his body.

Dermatitis from Canary Feathers

The case of 45-year-old Lewis R. was one of pure stubbornness.

Lewis' first trip to the physician's office was not his first experience with the ugly, itching rash that covered his face and arms. This first visit merely represented

Mrs. R.'s first successful attempt to induce her husband to investigate the cause of the rash.

Although the irritation seemed obviously to be the result of a contact irritant, the physician checked first on the foods. Finding nothing significant, he continued with the tests for contact irritants, but nothing appeared. A similar result with the bacterial group convinced the doctor that there was some detective work to be done.

"How often does this rash appear?" the physician asked.

"I can hardly say that it ever disappears," answered the patient. "There are some days when it seems to be worse than others."

"It is quite obvious, then, that whatever is irritating your skin must be constantly present. In that case, I must find out about everything you come into contact with regularly. It may be wise for me to visit your home," explained the physician.

Mr. R. exchanged glances with his wife. "Oh, I don't think that will be necessary," said Mr. R. boldly.

"I hope not but, if new evidence doesn't show up, I'll have no other alternative."

With this, the doctor referred to the autobiographical history of the case as obtained during the initial consultation, and questioned Mr. R. in detail about each individual point.

All through this tedious questioning, Mr. and Mrs. R. constantly exchanged those cryptic glances.

"Mr. R.," the doctor began after several silent moments, "if I'm to help you, I'll need your full cooperation. Are you sure there isn't something you have overlooked? Something you may have forgotten to tell me?"

"Not that I know of," Lewis said hesitantly.

"Then," began the doctor with an air of finality, "there is only one thing left for me to do. I'll have to come to your home and see for myself."

Mr. R.'s reaction indicated that he was not anxious for the doctor to come to his home. He was momentarily silent, then suddenly: "That's all right with me, Doctor, but, if you think I'll give up my canaries, you are mistaken," he warned.

The physician laughed. "Let's cross that bridge when we come to it. You hadn't told me about a canary, even though I asked whether you had any pets."

"Well, canaries aren't exactly pets," Lewis explained.

The physician's visit to his patient's home revealed that the man had not one or two canaries, but 40 of them in all parts of the house.

Mr. R. had felt all along that the birds were causing his trouble, but, like so many people, he could not bear to face the problem squarely. Raising canaries was his hobby, and what person likes to be told that his hobby is ruining his health?

A minimum of testing proved conclusively that the constant presence of canary dander in the air was the cause of the rash.

The irony of the whole case lies in the fact that it took the physician days to persuade Mr. R. to get rid of the birds in the interest of his own health. Uncomfortable and unpleasant as the ailment was to the man, he was not easily persuaded.

Today, less than year after sacrificing his hobby, Lewis R. is no longer ashamed of his appearance, for his rash has cleared up completely. His hobby? Well, he now derives a great deal of pleasure from writing authoritative articles on canaries for the various bird publications, as well as from collecting photographs of these birds.

Dermatitis from Goat Hair

Christmas had brought joy—and pain—to five-year-old Mary Lou. Under the Christmas tree stood that big rocking horse she had ordered from the department store Santa Claus.

It was a beautiful toy, and, for the first few days, Mary Lou spent most of her time on it. On the evening of the third day, the child complained about an itching sensation about her thighs and her backside. The frightened mother learned, after calling the physician, that Mary Lou was sensitive to the goat hair of which the rocking horse was made. Mary Lou reluctantly parted with her rocking horse, and the itching sensation disappeared.

CHAPTER

13 Urticaria and Angioedema

THESE CONDITIONS are essentially the same, except that urticaria, or small hives, is on the surface of the skin and angioedema, or giant hives, involves the deeper layers of the skin, the mucous membranes and the joints. If the swelling occurs in the throat or larynx, there can be asphyxiation unless help is promptly obtained. An injection of adrenalin is needed at this time.

The two conditions may be present in the same person and are often due to the same allergens. It is accepted and known by scientists in this field that certain foods, inhaled substances and drugs will cause urticaria and angioedema. There are many cases in which the condition will persist for many years and the cause is subtle and difficult to find. We have found in a number of such individuals hidden foci of infection in the teeth, gall bladder and bowels. When the infection cleared, the person recovered. The nervous system has been strongly implicated and the removal of a stressing emotional problem seems to have helped overcome some of these problems. This is still open to considerable question, as no scientific evidence appears sufficiently conclusive in this regard. Intestinal worms can also be a cause.

It must be clear to the reader that the usual thorough and complete examination and exhaustive laboratory studies are necessary, if this troublesome and often serious problem is to be solved.

Giant Hives from Fish Glue

Four-year-old Danny C. was considerably put out about the whole matter. Daddy C. shrugged his shoulders and protested against the barrage of accusations pouring from his wife.

"I knew it! I told you so!" she kept repeating. "The right kind of a father would keep at least one eye on his child when he takes him fishing!"

"I'm telling you I did keep an eye on him," protested the father. "I kept both eyes on him, and I'm sure he didn't leave my side the whole afternoon."

"The boy's probably poisoned, that's what," exclaimed Mrs. C. as she turned little Danny's face down on the bed for the tenth time. The left half of the child's backside had swollen to three times its normal size.

"It can't be poisoning," retorted the father. "I've fished that river for nearly 10 years, and I know there isn't a sign of poison ivy or poison oak for miles."

The family doctor looked at the inflamed region, then pressed it gently while the owner of the region indicated his disapproval.

"It's poisoning; I just know it is," said Mrs. C.

"I don't think so," ventured the doctor after a brief hesitation.

"Couldn't be a snake bite, could it, Doctor?" asked Mr. C.

"I'm sure it isn't that," replied the doctor. "Tell me —did anything unusual happen to the boy while he was with you? Did he do anything at all outside of sitting beside you?"

Mr. C. reflected. "Not that I remember."

At that moment, Danny flipped around to rest upon the unaffected portion of his backside and muttered something about being bitten by a fish. Daddy and mother were perfectly willing to pass it off as insignificant, but the doctor was interested.

"What do you mean, Danny?" inquired the physician.

"I spill itty fishes all over," he said cryptically.

"Oh, I know what he's talking about now," chuckled the father. "One time I asked him to push the minnow pail closer to me. He was so anxious that he pushed it over."

"Did any of the minnows spill out?" asked the doctor.

"Huh, just about every one of them," said the father. "Did manage to salvage a few, though."

The physician pieced the story together, made close examinations and smiled.

"Well, the boy has neither been poisoned nor bitten by a snake."

"Then what did happen to him?" the parents asked simultaneously.

"He sat on a minnow," replied the doctor.

"He what?" exclaimed the parents.

"Yes, he sat on a minnow," the doctor repeated. "You'll recall that, when Danny was still nursing, I had to eliminate fish from your diet, Mrs. C? Well, it seems that the child hasn't outgrown that sensitivity to fish. When he sat on that minnow, the glue on the scales worked its way into his pores, causing the reaction you see."

This "fish story" came to a happy ending when the swelling subsided, and the parents bent all their efforts toward keeping Danny away from fish in any form.

For those of you who are inclined toward practical joking, there is a sound lesson to be learned from the following episode in the life of a certain young lady.

Helen F. would have made a perfect hypochondriac

except for the fact that the ailments she constantly complained of actually existed.

When Helen said she had a pain in her side, she really had one. When she complained of a heart murmur or of a sudden loss of breath, there was a genuine foundation for the complaint. Her greatest fault was that she persisted in voicing her ailments to her friends. Even her best friends tired of it. Her friends tried ineffectually to talk her out of her complaints, but, when Helen said that a certain food was not good for her, she meant it. The gravity of the situation somehow did not impress others.

Helen belonged to a bridge club which met weekly. The girls had always respected Helen's request to eliminate certain foods from the luncheons they prepared.

One week, one of the girls was in the mood for practical joking.

"I'll bet it's all in her head," she told another member of the club. "I'll bet we could feed her crab meat, tell her it was tuna fish and she'd never know the difference."

"Why don't you try it?" suggested the other.

"That's exactly what I'm going to do. Won't Helen feel silly after we have told her that she has eaten crab meat?"

The girls arrived for their weekly meeting. As the luncheon was served several pairs of eyes focused with inconspicuous anxiety upon the unsuspecting Helen as she raised the first forkful of crab meat, alias tuna fish, to her lips. Since there was no immediate reaction, the girls believed that, for once, they were right.

Another mouthful and another, and suddenly Helen dropped her fork. The color left her cheeks as her lips turned blue. A terrified glassiness appeared in her eyes and, for a moment, silence hung over the room.

Soon Helen went into convulsions. She could not breathe. First aid was administered until a physician arrived. After an hour or so, Helen began to show indications of returning to normal. Only the use of adrenalin had kept the girl's heart beating.

Angioedema of the Larynx and Death

Mrs. Avis R., a patient of ours with bronchial asthma, tells us of her daughter's death at sixteen years of age. The story was substantiated by an autopsy report she furnished us. Her daughter had since two and a half years of age suffered from periodic swellings of a foot, a hand or the face following the eating of pork. One day at noon when she was sixteen years of age she ate some hot dogs in a restaurant. She was baby sitting and called her mother at 3:00 P.M. at which time she complained of laryngitis (hoarseness). At 9:00 P.M. that night she ran to a neighboring house dying of suffocation. Before medical attention could be obtained the youngster passed on. The autopsy report proved the death to be the result of asphyxiation due to swelling of the larynx caused by an allergic reaction. No doubt this was precipitated by pork which was contained in the hot dogs eaten at noon. Her mother knew that she ate nothing else between noon and the 3:00 P.M. telephone call. This tragedy might have been averted if the true nature of this girl's allergic problem had been understood and allergic medical consultation had been given many years earlier.

CHAPTER

14 *Digestive Allergy*

THIS IS KNOWN also as gastrointestinal allergy, and disturbances may show up from the mouth to the anus. The reaction may vary from mild to severe, and may include canker sores, nausea, vomiting and ulcerlike symptoms. There can be abdominal swelling with acute symptoms of pain, which may be localized to one area, such as the appendix, or there may be generalized discomfort. There is either constipation or diarrhea and a spastic colon or mucous colitis and general lassitude or allergic intoxication.

The causes usually are foods, but bacteria, intestinal parasites, drugs and even inhalants can cause or aggravate the conditions. Although these facts have been proved repeatedly and conclusively, there is still great reluctance in recognizing this fact, and individuals suffer needless discomfort, since they are often told that their problems are functional and due to nerves.

We have had instances of "ulcers" and mucous colitis in which proper study and food elimination produced complete "cures" after 9 to 15 years of suffering.

Allergy must be seriously considered in all digestive disturbances when no organic findings are disclosed. The examination is not concluded by simply stating that the condition is not organic and, therefore, that we have nothing to worry about. A thorough study must include a careful evaluation of other existing allergies and laboratory tests for special cells found in the blood stream and stools. Although skin tests are not

foolproof, they may reveal many items which can cause
difficulty. Though they may be only 50 per cent accurate, they still can help solve half the problems. The
use of a daily diary and trial diets will help us solve
this type of allergy.

Oli A. was 57 years old but, for most of her life, she
had so many symptoms that she had long since been
labeled a hypochondriac. She had been a sickly child
with recurring attacks of vomiting every few weeks.
She had been treated by her family physician 50 years
before. He had diagnosed an "exudative diathesis,"
because, in addition to the vomiting, she had recurring
attacks of "running" nose and chronic cough. She was
fortunate that, after several years, her troubles partially
subsided. Although she was of moderate build, her
weight was always below normal.

Fourteen years ago, she had brought her son to us
with severe bronchial asthma. He was 18 when we first
saw him. He was treated for asthma, is now a physician
himself and has been free of asthma for 10 years. Nine
years ago, Oli developed severe abdominal cramps and
hospitalization was required. Complete studies showed
no unusual organic findings. The condition was diagnosed as psychoneurosis with conversional symptoms in
her large bowel. She remained under the care of an excellent "stomach" specialist for all these years, when
it was suggested that her condition might be an allergy.
She remembered the successful treatment of her son's
asthma and came to us.

After a careful and complete history, physical examination and laboratory and allergy tests with special
food diaries and diets, we concluded that Oli had had
allergy most of her life and her large bowel was the
latest organ to become involved. She was found to be
highly allergic to milk and all milk products, wheat

and eggs. In addition, she was allergic to some of the bacteria from her colon (large bowel).

Within four months, she gained 18 pounds (from 97 pounds to 115 pounds). She lost her abdominal pains and her nervous condition improved remarkably. It is, of course, a new experience for Oli A. and it was needless for her to have suffered for so many years.

This is one of many cases of gastrointestinal or digestive allergy in our files. Cases of ulcer, chronic constipation, "heartburn," cyclic vomiting and others have been found to be due to allergy.

15 Drug and Chemical Allergies

DUE TO THE large number of new drugs which have been developed in the last 20 years, the problem of drug allergies has become very important. It is very important to understand that being allergic or hyper-sensitive to a particular drug is not the same as an intolerance to a drug or having a peculiar reaction to the toxic effects of the drug. The allergic reaction to a drug must be specific for a given drug and only after that drug has been previously taken without a reaction. For example, an aspirin tablet may cause ringing or buzzing in the ears of certain individuals; this would represent a peculiar reaction or idiosyncracy to the drug. If, however, an attack of asthma, or hives or a skin rash occurs, that is a drug allergy. One of the allergies must result from a reaction to a drug.

The types of allergic reactions seen from drugs are the sudden, severe or immediate type, known also as an anaphylactic reaction, in which shock may occur. This has occurred from an injection of penicillin or tetanus antitoxin (serum) and vitamin B, or from taking barbiturate drugs, penicillin, quinine, asprin or sulfa drugs. The danger here is that the tongue or voice box may be so swollen in giant hives that asphyxiation may result. This is known as angioedema.

The delayed type of reaction to drugs will frequently result after the first exposure to a drug. After about a week, the patient will begin to ache all over, have fever and swollen glands and break out with hives. Often, the joints become swollen and painful. This type of reaction is known as serum sickness. The rash can also be of the scaly type on areas which resemble black and blue marks (purpura). This condition has resulted from drugs, penicillin, sulfa, iodine, arsenic, gold, quinine, salicylates and barbiturates.

To those of you who read this book: if you have an allergy to *any* drug, be certain that you have this information in some obvious place on your person, as *it could be a matter of life or death*. In the following cases, this is illustrated.

Drug Allergy from Arsenic

Janet C., a 29-year-old woman with bronchial asthma for most of her life, sought relief by every means and traveled far and wide, until she finally entered a "special asthma clinic" where the sole treatment consisted of a cursory three-day examination and a bottle of medicine which was to cure her of asthma. Strange as it may seem, she did receive some relief from this liquid.

During a six-week period of ingesting this medication, her outlook improved, but this was soon to be followed by near disaster. She began to complain of itching of her skin. This became intense, and her entire body turned red and soon developed large blisters. She was now acutely ill; her skin began to peel in large flakes. Intensive treatment with intravenous medication, including ACTH and cortisone, saved her life. The medication she had been taking, it was learned, contained arsenic, to which she became extremely allergic. A very positive patch test proved it. The moral is do not take medication unless it is prescribed by

someone you can discuss your problem with, never take
it by remote control.

Chemical Allergy from Sodium Dichromate

Mary G. was 52, but had taken care of the cleaning in
the offices on the sixth floor of the Harding Building
for as long as she could remember. Recently, she developed a marked, generalized itchy skin eruption
which was getting worse; finally, she had to stop her
work. When she was seen, she required relief from the
itching since she had not slept for at least two weeks.
She was given medication for relief, and the acute condition subsided. Mary, however, had to work, and her
condition promptly returned. She was again relieved of
her symptoms and, on this occasion, was carefully
queried about the beginnings of this rash, which was
very widespread and disabling.

She recalled that she never had any difficulty until a
firm of architects moved to her floor. There were blueprints and liquid solutions used in their preparation.
It was very simple to discover Mary's allergy with a one-
quarter-inch patch test with the chemical solution
which contained sodium dichromate. This was used in
fixing the blueprints. Within two hours, the patch had
to be removed because of the intense reaction on her
back. Thus was cleared up the mystery of Mary's rash.

Anaphylactic Shock from Black Dye
(Paraphenylenediamine)

An attempt to economize on shoes nearly proved
fatal to Frank H., who decided that, instead of buying
new fall shoes, he would have his summer whites dyed
black.

The job was a good one. It was impossible to tell that
the shoes had once been white. But along came an

autumn rain and Frank's shoes were soaked. Less than an hour later, the man collapsed and appeared dead. It took oxygen and heart-stimulating adrenalin to bring him around. The dye from the shoes had found Frank's weakness. This should be the first substance suspected in cases of contact eruptions under dark clothing or furs.

CHAPTER

16 *Allergy from Fungus Infections*

THIS TYPE of allergy not infrequently follows an infection with one of the various fungi on the skin, and is due to the reaction of the fungi and the resulting substances entering the blood stream. The person with athlete's foot or ringworm of the scalp which may have persisted for many years may suddenly develop a rash elsewhere on the body. This may be similar to the focus of infection in a tooth with a resulting pain in a joint such as the shoulder or knee. The allergy has become apparent after the initial focus has been present for a period of time, producing the skin rash only after a new infection occurs. This has been proved scientifically and the conditions have been called by the original name with "id" added to it (trycophytid, epidermophytid and so forth) .

This condition frequently is due to neglect of the primary fungus infection or due to incorrect or too vigorous treatment, with resultant irritation. The use of strong local medication, or even X-ray treatment, added to the friction and maceration from strong soaps will cause this allergy. This can be demonstrated by a skin test to the fungus involved; it is usually very accurate. The hands and feet are most commonly involved in both the primary infection and the "id."

To establish the diagnosis is a relatively easy matter. This can be done by taking scrapings from the skin and examining them under the microscope. The hairs, scales of the skin, scrapings from nails and small skin blisters will usually, on examination, reveal the nature of the fungus involved in the primary disease. If any question remains, a culture of the material will reveal the culprit.

The treatment is good today. It was not always so, but, in recent years, the discovery of oral antifungus medication has made a difference. This, however, will not do the job alone; recurrence will result if the primary focus in the skin is not properly treated. All clothing, especially socks and shoes, must be adequately disinfected. In some cases, it may still be necessary to give allergic treatment in addition to the above, if one of the allergic skin conditions, such as contact dermatitis or atopic dermatitis, is present.

In order to round out this matter of contact irritants, we cannot overlook the molds as a source of sensitivity.

It would be simple, but useless, for us to spring upon the reader such names as *Cephalosporium* or *Trichophyton cerebriform*, and no doubt we'd have you worried. It is much less academic to explain that molds are those fuzzy growths that grow on bread, on the backs of books or, in fact, just about anywhere that bacteria do not grow. They require very little nourishment, but considerable dampness.

You can be certain that, wherever you are, the air and ground about you are saturated with many of the 265 kinds of mold spores known by scientists. If it will clarify this statement, we would like to say further that one tiny gram of soil has been found to contain 129,-000 such fungus spores.

Molds are the basis of such foods as cheese and yeast. Individuals found to be sensitive to such foods are merely reacting to the molds contained in them.

The thing to be remembered is that each mold spore is a living organism, and that anything living, whether it be a mother-in-law or a piece of yeast, is apt to cause an irritation if the right conditions exist.

You may have heard your doctor say that a bad tooth is a focus of infection. He simply means that, whatever your trouble is—arthritis, asthma or any other altered reaction—it originates in the bacterial or fungus infection around that bad tooth. Your difficulty could also have its origin in the tonsils, sinuses, bowels or genital area, for these are common foci of infection of bacteria or fungi.

17 *Allergy of the Eyes*

THE STRUCTURES of the eye are frequently involved with allergy. Symptoms such as smarting, burning, itching or thickening of the eyelids may be mild or can be very serious, involving the eyeball and inner structures of the eye. Ulceration, cataracts and even blindness can occur. Allergy of the eyes, in most cases, can be cured or marked relief can be obtained, if patience, proper allergic study and good eye care are given.

Among the frequent conditions affecting the eye, contact dermatitis of the lids is probably the most common and the least serious. The skin will thicken, wrinkle and discolor due to the rubbing because of the itching. In women, the causes are usually cosmetics. In men, the usual causes are shaving materials, hair tonics, tobacco or some occupational contact.

The cause must be found and removed early or complications will result by affecting the lining of the eyeball proper or conjunctiva. This will cause congestion, watering of the eyes and extreme light sensitivity, requiring the use of sunglasses.

Angioedema of the eye structures, as in other cases of giant hives, is due to bedding, feather pillows, woolen coverings or face creams.

A condition known as blepharitis involves the edge or margin of the eyelids with congestion, scales and, at times, weeping. This is often due to cosmetics. It is frequently associated with dandruff of the scalp, which may aggravate the condition. To cure the allergy, the scalp must be treated for dandruff. Staphylococci are responsible for some of these conditions because the individual has become allergic to these bacteria.

Sties and cysts about the eyelids, if other causes are eliminated, may be due to food allergens, inhalants and staphylococci.

Conjunctivitis is common as an allergic manifestation, and may be due to most external allergens. Extreme itching, burning, tearing and light-sensitiveness, as well as spasms about the eyes, are common. The lids will reveal pinpoint- to pin-head-sized hives. The lower lid is usually the more seriously affected. The most severe forms of conjunctivitis are known as vernal catarrh. Conjunctivitis is commonly associated with the respiratory allergies, hay fever, perennial allergic rhinitis and asthma.

The conditions involving the deeper structures, such as the cornea, lens, retina and others, are too technical to be satisfactorily presented, but they are involved in the problem of allergy. If a condition persists after the usual treatment, one must consider the possibility of an allergic cause. Cataracts, gradual loss of vision and near-sightedness have not infrequently been associated with allergy.

A sudden loss of vision from excessive smoking or the taking of alcoholic beverages is due to allergy to the grain or tobacco leaf, or to sensitivity to alcohol, respectively. There are many such cases on record.

18 *Allergic and Migraine Headaches*

HEADACHES ASSOCIATED with hay fever, perennial allergic rhinitis and many of the eye allergies are common. These headaches are usually secondary to the primary allergic condition, and are cured when the primary allergy is corrected.

There are certain headaches which are due to hypersensitivity. One type with which most people are familiar is the migraine headache, which leaves the victim exhausted, tense and fearful of its recurrence. Approximately 11 per cent of the typical migraine headaches are due to allergy. Allergic headaches have been "cured" by the avoidance of a single food allergen when it has been discovered as the cause.

It is extremely important to understand that a person with headaches should be thoroughly evaluated from the standpoint of physical defects, such as defective vision, high blood pressure, kidney disease, anemia, emotional states and the presences of surgical conditions in the ears, eyes, nose and throat. Laboratory and X-ray studies, including angiograms of the blood vessels of the skull and brain for possible tumor or disease, should be done. With completely normal findings from this type of investigation, we can then certainly complete the study by a thorough allergic study, subsequent management and care. (This will be elaborated in Part III of this book.) It is quite clear that certain headaches have both allergic and physical factors. Under such circumstances, it is necessary to cor-

rect both conditions. There are headaches which so
closely resemble the migraine or allergic headaches
that only the most subtle and skillful evaluation can
arrive at a correct diagnosis. The clue may have been
present only for a very short time early in the patient's
life. A marked sensitivity to one food, such as egg, which
caused vomiting may be the key which will open a
recalcitrant lock.

Although foods are usually the allergens causing
allergic headache, it is necessary to remove all inhalant
and other allergens as well as to lighten the total burden
which might trigger the headache. Removal of the
foods or building the patient's resistance by injections
against the offenders, rigid adherence to diet and environmental control of inhalant factors, along with
adequate rest, good bowel habits and correction of
all other physical defects, are all of extreme importance.
The two cases which follow very dramatically illustrate
the benefits of careful allergic study and treatment.

This is the tale of a headache severe as an Artic
blizzard and regular as the sunrise. The headache belonged to a dignified spinster in her late forties.

For several years, she had visited physicians of all
kinds, hoping that she would learn the cause of her
headaches and whether or not she could ever expect
to be rid of them. After exhausting her list of general
practitioners, she started down the list of specialists,
and although she did not expect that she would need
a brain operation, the woman, Ellen B., headed her
list with a brain specialist.

There were many questions and quite a thorough
examination of the brain, but this specialist concluded
that the headache was probably migraine, inherited
from her mother.

Not having remembered her mother, Miss B. had

no reason to doubt this diagnosis, but, since the physician offered no constructive advice, she also had little reason to believe that her trouble was migraine. Accordingly, she went to see an eye, ear, nose and throat man.

A thorough examination of these organs convinced her that the difficulty was not here.

Next came the dentist, who agreed that a localized reaction such as her headache might very likely originate in the teeth. Searching for a focus of infection, he found, to his surprise, that Ellen B. possessed a perfect set of teeth. Infection? There wasn't even a slight cavity.

Miss B. decided to reason the thing out further. A headache, she figured, must have something to do with nerves. Searching everywhere, she finally located a neurologist with a fine reputation.

There were, of course, a lot of new questions along with a repetition of the old ones. The neurologist concluded that there must be an inflamed nerve in that particular part of her head that ached.

Since it was impossible to remove the nerve, the next best thing to do was to strengthen the entire nervous system. The task fell to vitamin B-1 and Ellen B. gave the vitamins a fair chance. After several months, she was convinced that there was no improvement.

She was X-rayed, fluoroscoped and examined in every way possible, but the doctors simply threw in the sponge, while the patient continued to suffer through her excruciating headaches. It began to appear as though the migraine theory was right. Just about the time Miss B. had decided that her headache was there to stay, someone suggested the name of a physician who had been known to trace the source of headaches through skin tests.

Feeling that she had nothing to lose, Miss B. visited

this new type of specialist, who sat patiently and listened to each little detail with great interest, requesting elaboraion of each apparenly insignificant point.

"You say your headache appears regularly every Tuesday morning?" asked the doctor.

Ellen B. assured him of this.

"And how does it affect you?" he asked.

"I only know that the pain is unbearable," replied Miss B. "When I feel the headache coming on, there is nothing I can do but to take a sleeping potion and go to bed."

"Does this help to eliminate the ache?"

"I don't believe it does. It merely makes me less conscious of it."

"How long do the headaches last?" asked the doctor.

"They have lasted as long as three days, but they generally start to wear off by the end of the second day."

The physician began to administer the skin tests but found that group after group registered negatively. If there were only one tiny reaction, he thought, there would be something to work on.

The doctor's patience was rewarded. On the seventieth test, there showed a strong reaction to garlic. The doctor looked at his patient. She was a dignified sort of person whom one just didn't associate with garlic. Perhaps the reaction wasn't related. But then, perhaps it was. Miss B. was paying good money to find out, and there was nothing to do but follow up the clue.

"Miss B," he began, as tactfully as possible, "do you care for spicy food?"

"Not especially," was the reply. "Oh—with one exception," she added, grinning sheepishly. "Just between us, I'm very fond of garlic."

"And do you cook with it often?" asked the physician.

"Not often. You see, I meet many friends and people socially, and must not eat garlic-flavored foods for this reason. But, one evening a week, I treat myself. Monday evening, I always prepare a thick, juicy steak with garlic rubbed over it," she explained.

The doctor smiled. "You are evidently not aware of the fact that you have practically diagnosed your own case," he said.

"You mean that my headaches are caused by plain, simple garlic?" she asked.

"We have merely to confirm it," stated the doctor. "I want you to deviate from your routine. Although this is not Monday, I should like you to buy that thick, juicy steak, rub it with garlic and prepare it for this evening's dinner. Then I want you to phone me immediately if you have a recurrence of your headache tomorrow morning."

Miss B. followed her instructions, and the next morning the physician received the call he had hoped for. The headache had returned.

A reverse procedure was followed in which garlic was strictly eliminated from the patient's diet for a period of two months. During that time, she hadn't been troubled with a single headache. Then came one more dose of garlic for further verification, and when the headache reappeared, the case was closed.

Miss B. has completely and conscientiously eliminated this spice from her diet, and she has spent two years without the discomfort of her former ailment.

In order that you may not come to the logical, but erroneous, conclusion that all these so-called unusual ailments are simple afflictions that are easily and painlessly diagnosed, the following case is related."*

*This case is from the files of Alfred M. Goltman, M.D., of Memphis, Tennessee (now deceased).

A young woman, as in the previous case, was troubled with severe headaches. She, too, had made the rounds of the specialists, but without results.

Having eventually arrived at the physician's office for skin tests, she admitted that there wasn't anything she would refuse to do, if she could just rid herself of the perennial headache.

The young lady, whom we'll call Mary D., meant precisely what she said, for her headache endured ceaselessly for nearly one year. To a great extent, it had colored her behavior. Mary's particular weakness was a serious one—wheat. We say serious because it is difficult to build an attractive diet on foods that do not contain wheat.

Through various medical examinations, it was proved that her headaches were caused by pressure within the skull due to swollen brain membranes. The doctor conferred with several brain specialists who unanimously confirmed this diagnosis.

There was only one way to prove it, and Mary D. was consulted. The physicians wanted permission to cut away a small portion of her skull so as to expose the brain to view. They would then give her concentrated injections of wheat to observe the reaction of the brain at the point of opening.

Miss B. agreed to the operation, and the skull was opened precisely at the region where the headaches occurred.

"Incredible!" exclaimed the doctors simultaneously when they noted the reaction of the wheat injections. The membranes of the brain had swollen to the point of protruding through the opening in the skull. Then, when the effects wore off, the membranes shrank back to their normal position.

The experiment was carried on for several days in order to verify the results, and each time the wheat caused the same reaction.

The next question was what to do about it. We could not build a reception room on the side of her head to accommodate the expanding portion of her brain, but, as long as the girl stayed away from wheat in any of its forms, she was not troubled. She had a rigid list of food restrictions, and, as soon as she was well enough, immunization against wheat was begun.

CHAPTER

19 *Insects and Allergy*

INSECTS CAN cause allergy in one of three ways: by inhalation of scales or dusts from the wings and body, by injection of the venom through the sting or by the instillation of salivary secretion.

It is well known that many of us fail to react very much to the bite of a specific insect. On the other hand, a severe reaction can occur. This is not due to the irritant material, but rather to an acquired sensitivity. There have been as many as 30 different insects listed in our medical literature as having caused allergic symptoms. As early as 1811, a case of bee sensitivity is recorded.

Some of the insects that commonly cause allergic symptoms are the caddis fly, May fly, wasp, flea, bedbug, mosquito, horsefly, citrus fruit fly, beetle, bee, ant, moths and yellow jacket.

The allergy from insects is usually a large local swelling, but it may be all over the body in the form of stinging, burning and smarting hives. If the sensitivity is severe, it can cause asthma, with swelling of the throat, shortness of breath, coughing and tightness of the chest. If the reaction is stronger, it can result in a severe general reaction with shock and collapse and death. All these reactions may occur within a few minutes to a few hours. Children seem somewhat more susceptible than adults, and they usually develop skin allergies, such as hives, often associated with infection because of the scratching from the severe itching.

Deaths which have been recorded have been caused by the bee, wasp, ant and hornet. Severe reactions have been recorded from moths and caterpillars, mosquitoes, yellow jacket, aphids, housefly, fleas, bedbugs and gnats. Scorpions and spiders, though not insects, can cause serious reactions.

Certain preventive measures may be used for treatment, especially of skin allergies from insects. A spray of 5 per cent DDT will kill most insects and prevent symptoms. Dr. Harvey Blank, in 1950, suggested the following procedure for the prevention of contact with insects.

(a) Apply 5 per cent DDT (r) on dogs, cats and under cushions and rugs and avoid contact with these pets. This is also of value for mosquitoes, fleas and bedbugs.

(b) Dust the individual with the powder lightly, and include the bed clothes and mattress.

(c) Care should be taken to avoid contaminating foods, dishes and cooking utensils. Air the room after spraying.

(d) Wipe excess spray from pets with a damp cloth to keep them from eating the powder.

(e) Make sure that there is a light film of powder on the individual and that the spray contains 5 per cent DDT.

Insect repellents are effective if adequately and uniformly distributed, but they may irritate the skin and are harmful to eyes and toxic when taken internally. Most repellents are solvents of many paints, varnishes and plastics and may damage plastic materials, but will not damage wool clothing. They are applied to the skin, with a few drops in the hands smeared evenly on all exposed skin. For ant control, sodium arsenite mixed with ample sugar syrup or chlordane is very

effective. Stings of the bee, hornet, wasp, yellow jacket
and ant should be considered as serious and emergent,
and promptly treated by your physician with adrenalin, 1—1000 solution, 0.5 cc. by injection. A few drops
of adrenalin may be injected into the bite. This will
contract the blood vessels and delay the absorption
into the blood stream. Antihistamines may be given
intravenously and by mouth. One may be selected from
those listed under drugs in allergy. For spider and scor-
pion bites, your doctor may give calcium gluconate and
magnesium sulphate intravenously into the blood
stream. Local treatment is of no great benefit in serious
reactions.

The skin test study of the insect-sensitive patient
must include a sufficient variety of all possible insects
known to cause allergic symptoms. The insect allergens
used must be potent; they must have been scientifically
prepared and tested. The history of previous contact
with insects, such as beekeepers or those whose hobby
may be insects, might be of great value in evaluating
the study. Other associated allergies may have to be
considered in the entire picture, if complete benefit of
treatment is to be obtained. When the specific insect is
incriminated by allergic skin tests, injections by hyposensitizing the individual to the insect are usually very
successful. Prevention, of course, by screens and insecticides should be seriously worked on.

Through the following example, some of this discussion will be more clearly understood. Delay in treatment may be serious.

Insect Allergy from Bee Stings

Jim B., a handsome, well-built man of 42 years of
age, was very nervous and appeared visibly apprehen-
sive. Only 24 hours before, he had been unconscious

and narrowly escaped death. He was saved, thanks to his clear-thinking wife and the fortunate coincidence that the family doctor was next door seeing a patient. Dr. Smith correctly sized up the situation, administered a large dose of adrenalin into the vein and treated Jim for shock. Soon, his color, breath and pulse began to return, and, within minutes, he sat wondering what hit him, although he really knew the answer.

Jim is a captain of a large jet airliner, and, a few years ago, took up honeybees as a hobby. Recently, he had noted a change in his reaction to the bee sting, for he had been stung many times previously. The first time his changed reaction expressed itself in swelling at the site of the sting, with some numbness of the hand and arm. The second time he had a similar reaction, but with the addition of some hives and itching over his entire body, some shortness of breath and marked weakness. Dr. Smith was called, he gave him adrenalin and warned him to see an allergist who would study and treat him, for the next time it could be fatal. He did not go to the specialist. His third experience was almost his last.

Study revealed that he was allergic to bees, hornets and wasps. He also had some minor allergic manifestations, such as frequently recurring, but not disabling, coughs and colds due to household dusts. Treatment for the insects and dust has placed Jim in a good state of allergic balance, and he no longer worries about his problem. As a pilot, with so many lives in his care, this is a must for Jim.

CHAPTER
20 Miscellaneous Allergies

BY THIS TIME, it must be clear that practically every organ or tissue of the human body can become hypersensitive and be the site of an allergic reaction.

Most of us have come to know the common allergies, such as bronchial asthma, hay fever, perennial allergic rhinitis, atopic dermatitis, most forms of contact dermatitis, urticaria, angioedema and digestive disturbances. It is not so well known that allergy can cause certain nervous disorders, including Ménière's disease, convulsions, pain, bleeding and colicky spasms of the kidneys, bladder and urinary tract; bleeding into the skin and mucous membranes called purpura; severe menstrual cramps and discharge; some forms of joint disease and arthritis and certain conditions of the mouth, throat, eyes and ears. Physical allergy to heat, cold and light are also included. Allergy can be strongly suspected in these conditions, when thorough examinations have revealed no other cause and when the patient has demonstrated allergy either present or past. A strong family history of allergy is highly significant in making a diagnosis of allergy.

Nervous allergy has, in recent years, received considerable attention. Although no set personality pattern has been found to exist in the allergic person, there are some strong suggestions that they are frequently hyperirritable. The electroencephalogram has, in some instances, shown alterations in children, especially those with behavior problems.

Epilepsy has been regarded as an allergic disease by some allergists, and a small percentage is due to allergy. Foods appear to be the most likely cause, although all factors must be considered and the evaluation must be most thorough.

Multiple sclerosis has recently been studied along allergic lines. The allergen causing the condition may be within the body. It has been difficult to prove at the present time, but, again, if suspected, the most painstaking studies of all medical factors should be done before an allergic survey is undertaken.

Uterus, kidney and bladder allergy is not a rarity. Colic from kidney spasms, frequency of urination with bleeding, dysmenorrhea and uterine cramps have occurred from inhaling pollens or the ingestion of foods. Injections of various allergens have produced symptoms by causing irritation and bleeding of the mucous membrane and colic from the muscle spasms of the uterus or bladder. The swelling and irritation in these organs and tissues resembles many other conditions affecting the genitourinary system.

Purpura has been seen frequently from hypersensitivity to foods, drugs or inhaled allergens. This bleeding into the skin may be accompanied by gastrointestinal symptoms such as nausea, vomiting, abdominal cramps and diarrhea and, often, arthritis. This condition is known as Henock's or Schönlein's-Henock's syndrome. It must again be called to the attention of the reader that only if sufficient evidence is present to suspect allergy should such studies and management be carried out. Thorough medical studies should precede the allergic survey and management.

However, the sufferer should not permit negative medical findings to cause him to despair.

The allergic joint is not infrequently observed. It is known as intermittent hydrathrosis, and is often seen after a person, allergic to horse serum, has been given tetanus antitoxin. The joint will become painful and swollen, and fluid will accumulate in the joint space. Specific food allergy may also cause this condition. A complete cure may be accomplished by complete avoidance of the offending foods.

Rheumatoid arthritis has been suspected as being an allergy to bacteria, especially the streptococcus. It has also been interesting to note that many patients with rheumatoid arthritis have an allergic history. The allergic phase of the problem must be carefully and thoroughly investigated in these individuals.

Allergies of the mouth, throat and ears can be due to drugs, foods, contact from dentures and orthodontia devices. Other conditions that may cause soreness of the mouth and throat must be eliminated, such as infection in the mouth and teeth, which may also be a source of the sensitivity. General physical disease must be considered in such cases. Canker sores and herpes due to foods, spices and drugs are quite common. The allergy must be discovered if a "cure" is to be obtained. Vomiting is usually a manifestation of many gastrointestinal conditions, but it can be due to foods, especially in children, and can well be a forerunner of migraine headaches later in life. Deafness can be the result of an allergic process in the ear. It is due to swelling and accumulated fluid in the middle ear. All parts of the hearing apparatus may be swollen from the external ear canal to the eustachian tube in back of the throat. If the swelling is not reduced, infection, which will further aggravate the impaired hearing, can take place. This type of conductive deafness is the most common type of allergy of the ear.

There are a series of conditions called collagen diseases. They include rheumatic fever, rheumatoid arthritis, scleroderma, dermatomyositis and periarteritis nodosa, as well as several others. They are merely mentioned so the reader will know that, although they are considered hypersensitivity diseases, the allergy has not been clearly established so that it may be of practical use in treatment. Investigators have produced similar diseases in animals by the use of drugs and horse serum. It is well to know that we are making serious inroads into these one time hopeless diseases. The following pages will reveal interesting allergic problems that illustrate how varied the subject can be and clarify the fact that any tissue or organ of the body may be involved.

Those who didn't know Frank T. intimately thought he was the most fortunate creature alive. Not many men at the age of 40 were so successful in business. Not many men were able to retire at this age.

Those who did know Frank T. knew that, as a human dynamo, there wasn't anything in the world he wanted more than to be able to stay on the job.

He had no alternative. He had visited every prominent heart specialist in the country, but all he learned was that "a certain condition existed." Judging from the number of times Frank T. had lapsed into unconsciousness during recent years, it was apparent that a certain condition existed. But, regardless of the number of cardiographs taken, or of the number of fees paid for professional services, he invariably went home without knowing anything further about the ailment, why it existed or what could be done about it.

All the physicians prescribed rest, so Frank spent the

first year of his premature retirement resting. Much to
his disgust, he felt like a fifth wheel on a wagon. But,
worst of all, his condition had not improved.

The doctors agreed that his coma resembled death
more closely than anything they had ever witnessed,
but all they did was shrug their shoulders and send
Frank more statements.

Frank planned to explore the European field for new
cardiac specialists. There were several in Vienna, one
in Paris, one in Berlin and a couple in London.

Money was no object. If there was a cure, he wanted
it, even if it cost him his last million. The next trans-
atlantic liner carried him to the European specalists.
They, too, were convinced that a certain condition
existed, but were reluctant to venture further into the
matter.

To say the least, Frank T. was disconcerted. As he
traveled from one European city to the next, he ration-
alized that at least the scenery was beautiful even if the
doctors were unsatisfactory.

It all seemed hopeless, but Frank gave the Europeans
every opportunity to make good. He spent nearly three
years trying out the various spas and rest cures recommended by the doctors.

The Riviera was beautiful; the sunset on Lake
Lucerne was gorgeous and a small picturesque resort
buried away in southern France was peaceful and color-
ful. What's more, the chef there was a master in the art
of barbecuing pork over an open fire.

Frank's condition refused to respond to this treatment. As a matter of fact, he found that his spells
occurred more often. His thoughts wandered back to
his native land. He longed to hear the roar of the ele-
vated and the blast of automobile horns. He yearned
for the sight of a million people pouring into the sub-

ways at five o'clock. He wondered whether that hole-in-the-wall just off Broadway, near his office, still turned out the best pork sausage and pancakes in the city.

Frank T. made up his mind. As impulsively as he had gone to Europe, he returned to the United States. He had breakfast at the hole-in-the-wall, and then headed toward his family doctor's office.

Frank suddenly felt very ill. He recognized it as the beginning of a spell, but there wasn't anything he could do. He grew weak, then faint, and everything went blank.

He was in a drugstore when he regained consciousness. Standing over him were two men, obviously a pharmacist and a physician.

"You've had a close shave," said one of the men. "Don't be afraid. I just gave you an injection of adrenalin—heart stimulant, you understand."

Frank sat up. "You're telling me about adrenalin," he said. "It's been keeping me alive for six years."

Becoming interested, the doctor asked several questions. Frank answered all the questions and expected the customary diagnosis, "a certain condition." This time he was surprised for the physician went a step further.

"You have a certain unusual condition, and, if you come to my office, I rather believe that I can find out what's causing it."

Within three weeks, Frank's food tendencies were broken down. He was shocked to learn that those delicious pork sausages were his "poison." Enlightened, he then recalled that his spells at the resort in southern France occurred precisely on the evenings when the chef made those delectable pork roasts over the open fire.

Scientifically, his disorder was known as Ménière's disease. Acting as an irritant, the pork would cause a swelling of a brain nerve, then of the brain. The pressure created against his inner ears brought about the spells of coma.

Frank T. has been under strict diet restriction for over a year now, and has yet to suffer his first spell since swearing off pork.

Another interesting case was that of Lea B., a 14-year-old girl who suffered from rather large black and blue areas on the skin. About three and a half months before she consulted an allergist, Lea had been exposed to a high concentration of mineral spirits for at least three days. Within a week, she became nauseated and vomited bloody material. This was followed by painful joints, especially the hips and knees, and small hemorrhages in the skin. This condition was present most of the time, and became worse at times when there appeared to be blood in the urine and stools, with swelling of the face, feet and ankles. There were severe joint pains and small hives all over the body. This condition was persisting much too long so consultations were held.

Study revealed that allergy was strongly positive in the family, and that Lea also had her share of it as eczema and, later, hay fever, which was always worse during the Johnson and Bermuda grass season. It was of interest to note that, when she was a child, her father had been in the paint business and often cleaned brushes with mineral spirits. Her home was adjacent to the store, and the child played there most of the time.

Except for some kidney irritation and the trouble in her skin and joints, no serious blood diseases were found. After complete allergic study and management, in which a program of food avoidance, mainly of milk, eggs and fish, was instituted and hyposensitization to the grasses, dust and several other inhalants was begun, the black and blue skin areas began clearing, and all other symptoms subsided; complete recovery resulted.

When is a sore throat not a sore throat? Sounds like a foolish question, but there is a sensible answer, and the next case illustrates this fact.

The sore throat in question happened to Robert F., a domesticated young husband who felt quite at home in the kitchen. As a matter of fact, Robert's wife considered him a backseat cook of the most provoking type. For weeks, she had threatened a sit-down strike, but either Robert didn't scare easily or he didn't believe his wife would carry out her threat. Consequently, the backseat cooking continued until one day when the breaking point was reached Mrs. F. not only went on a strike, but she informed hubby that she was going to give him two or three weeks to get the culinary habit out of his system. She was going to visit her mother, and he would not only have to cook for himself, but also wash his own dishes.

It was this last blow that hurt, but hubby took it like a man, and did an amateur job of concealing disapproval.

With Mrs. F. away, Robert proceeded to prove that he could take care of himself. Aside from being lonesome, he didn't mind his situation. He could turn out a tasty meal.

It was on the second morning after Mrs. F.'s departure that Robert's sore throat appeared. He dismissed it with an "Oh, well," and proceeded to gargle hot salt water.

Taking a small bag of salt, a teaspoon and a tumbler to the office with him, he would gargle each hour, then swallow imaginary lumps to determine whether or not

the sore throat had improved. But, alas, it was just as
bad as ever, and now his tonsils were irritated by the
hot salt water.

At the end of the day, Robert went home, made
dinner and gargled before retiring. The next morning,
he awoke to find that he had not thrown off his malady, and so he repeated his hourly gargling for the
rest of the day. The sore throat was still there, although
it had shifted from the vicinity of his tonsils to a spot
inches deeper in his throat.

For the second day, Robert F. endured the agony
of a "galloping sore throat," but he kept his courage
as he went home and cooked his dinner for the third
evening. He had already decided that, if the next day
brought no improvement, he would have the family
doctor paint the throat with silver nitrate.

Twenty-four hours later, he made application for
the interior paint job.

"Strange thing about that sore throat," said the
doctor in a puzzled tone of voice. "It doesn't look like
an infection."

Twenty-four hours later, Robert F. returned to report that the silver nitrate might just as well have been
left in the bottle. The family physician wrapped up a
few pills and issued them to his patient with instructions. The patient would have agreed to anything if he
could only get rid of that sore throat; it made him feel
miserable.

Several more days passed. There was nobody to offer
Robert sympathy, for his sore throat had not departed.
He was increasingly a sadder man as he came home each
evening to make dinner.

By this time, he had taken matters into his own
hands. He had even tried painting his own throat with

a horrible-tasting antiseptic, but somehow he only seemed to "chase" the irritation from one region to another.

Several days later, Robert received a letter from his wife, telling him that she would be back in a few days. The news was great, except that, if he didn't rid himself of the sore throat, he'd never hear the end of it.

The thought upset him so that he worried all day. This brought a clear case of acid indigestion. Result: before cooking dinner that evening, he took some baking soda.

"Gosh!" he exclaimed, as he swallowed heavily three or four times. "It's gone!" Racing madly for the phone, he called the doctor to tell him the news.

"You mean that the soreness disappeared the moment the baking soda touched it?" repeated the doctor.

"Just as though it had never been sore," explained Mr. F. "What do you make of it?"

"Chemically speaking, you must have had an acid condition which was neutralized by the baking soda," replied the doctor. "Tell me, have you been eating very much of any one particular food since your throat became sore?"

"Well, yes," Robert said hesitatingly. "You see, I love pork sausage, but my wife refuses to make it very often because it is quite spicy. With her away for the past couple of weeks, I thought this was a good chance for me to have as much of it as I wanted. The day she left town, I bought five pounds of it, and I've had it for breakfast and dinner every day since," he admitted.

A visit to the doctor's office the next day proved conclusively to Robert F. that his body was extremely sensitive to pork. While he ate it occasionally, a toxic condition never existed. It was only after his continued diet of this particular food that the quantity became sufficient to bring about its manifestation.

"What you actually had," explained the doctor, "was a strawberry rash. Only it wasn't caused by strawberries, and it appeared in your throat, rather than on the outside of your body."

That the orthopedic physicians are becoming increasingly more aware of the existence of specific weakness in the human body is well exemplified by the following narrative.

Bobby W. was unofficially judged a perfect baby. When he was born, the pediatricians said they hadn't seen such a well-formed child in a long time. Bobby's parents were tickled pink. This meant that their son was, physically speaking, going to have an even chance to lick life.

Mother followed the doctor's orders and Bobby came along fine. The years slipped by, and there was a physical checkup every six months. Mrs. W. decided that this was the only way to learn of an ailment before it became serious.

Suddenly, at the age of eight, Bobby developed a limp in his right leg. The parents were worried, for infantile paralysis was prevalent in the county. Terror-stricken, Mrs. W. phoned for the doctor, who convinced her that the paralysis theory was out, although he wasn't quite certain of the nature of this ailment.

Within a few days, the limp had disappeared almost as abruptly as it had come. A week later it was back.

This time, the pediatrician referred Mrs. W. to an orthopedic physician, who X-rayed the child's bones and their connecting tissues. Here he noticed something unusual, for the tissue in the right hip joint was inflamed and obviously enlarged.

"Has the boy had any falls lately?' the doctor asked.

Mrs. W. convinced him that there had been none of a serious nature.

The physician was bewildered. Here was a case unlike any he had ever encountered. He X-rayed the hip joint regularly for the next five or six days, and saw the inflamed condition return to normal before his very eyes. Once again, the child was walking without a limp. Once again, the X-ray pictures showed absolutely nothing.

"I'd like you to get in touch with me if this thing happens again," the doctor requested of Mrs. W.

It wasn't until the next recurrence of the swollen hip joint that the orthopedic physician made up his mind to try a different angle. There had been previous instances in which testing for sensitivity through intramuscular injections had revealed the contributing factors.

"We're going to try something," he informed Mrs. W. "And I feel confident that, in a very short time, we shall know what is causing the trouble."

Bobby was taken to a specialist in skin-testing and diagnosis, who ran down the foods over a period of several weeks. Bobby showed a reaction to fish, and markedly to salmon. Further experimentation proved that, when the boy ate salmon, he developed a case of hives about his right hip joint. The joint, in turn, would swell, making it difficult for the boy to walk.

The strict elimination of salmon from the child's diet has, of course, done away with the annoying limp.

Then there was the unusual case of Mary D., who developed an irritating rash on her legs after being splashed with slush while waiting for a streetcar.

Hers was one of those rare cases of sensitivity toward weather which was treated by cool baths in which the

temperature of the water was lowered at regular intervals. Eventually, Miss D. immunized herself against
irritations from cold and dampness.

It is this same sensitivity toward temperature changes
that causes the shock known to bathers as "cramps,"
accountable for many drownings each year.

CHAPTER

21 *Some Psychosomatic Aspects of Allergy*

YOU HAVE just read two newspaper articles. One of them concerns an individual whom you do not know. You think: "So what?"

The second clipping concerns you, or a member of your family or, perhaps, a close friend. Well, now, that is a different story. You read and reread the item until you know practically every word of it from memory.

The point is that the degree of interest one takes in something is determined principally by the factor of proximity. In other words: "How close does this come to touching my own life?"

Look out of the nearest window. The man coming down the street is a total stranger. You've never seen him in your life. It is not unreasonable to expect that you are not the least bit interested in him or how his personality impresses others.

Look into the nearest mirror. The person you are looking at is the most interesting person in the world to you. That individual's personality and the manner in which it is projected to society are of utmost importance to you, because they are your own.

The person who is "disgustingly healthy" need consider only normal factors when determining his personality problem. The degree of positive or negative appeal he makes upon others can be controlled almost entirely through will power and the use of his mind.

Upon analyzing himself, a person of this type may come to realize that his strongest nagative characteristic is the fact that he speaks too loudly. With a certain amount of effort, he can curb this tendency.

Individuals with physical handicaps find themselves with an additional problem, even if they are otherwise healthy and normal.

Compensation is the term used by the psychologists. It is a gratifying substitute in interests when one is handicapped physically. The particular behavior of the blind or the crippled is colored by these factors. Consequently, the blind often resort to the use of their hands to compensate for their defect. The quantity, as well as the quality, of the work they can do is very often astounding.

Persons who have been deprived of the use of one or more limbs often develop very active minds. If they are shut-ins and are otherwise quite healthy, they may establish wide-reaching successful businesses right in their homes. Some have edited publications, others have carried on public secretarial services.

What happens to the individual who learns that he is slightly different from the average normal person because he happens to be allergically sensitive to certain substances? Perhaps, as in the case of Bill M. reviewed in this volume, the presence of pencil sharpener dust in the air brings on a constant attack of sneezing together with the sensation of smelling flowers.

Bill, as you will recall, has been ridiculed by his co-workers, and, consequently, his behavior is affected. He may have been nicknamed "Sneezy" or something equally embarrassing. The effect of this nickname upon Bill's dignity is devastating. As a result, he subconsciously develops a defense mechanism with which to combat the nickname. The defense mechanism may take the form of sarcasm, which, at times, may burn too deeply, further broadening the breach of relations between Bill and the jester.

If Bill finds himself obliged to defend his dignity, he may eventually become antagonistic to justify his being known as a "sourpuss."

As time marches on, Bill becomes adjusted to the characteristics involuntarily attached to him. His personality alters itself to correspond, and presently he finds himself projecting his office personality when he is out in society.

There is one morsel of gratification in the knowledge that, by using self-control, Bill M. need not disclose his weekday characteristics to new individuals entering his life. You see, his hypersensitivity to pencil dust has disrupted his normal and positive personality without altering his physical appearance.

What about the fellow who is not quite so fortunate? Susceptibility to certain irritants may make a visible change in appearance. Such a person is to be pitied, although pity, in itself, is hardly a treatment.

Yes, it happens to a number of Marys, Bettys, Bills, Georges and Freds, and it *may* happen to you. External manifestations of hypersensitivity are quite common, and, although they may not be serious in themselves, they present sights that are grossly misleading.

We have only to refer to such cases as the one in which the man went into a coma after eating pork, or that in which the child developed a nasty skin eruption from sitting upon a minnow or that in which the steel mill foreman's body was covered with a rash. These are illustrative of the thousands upon thousands of similar cases caused by as many different irritants.

These are the cases in which we find the truly pitiable and depressing stories. In many instances, those afflicted die a thousand deaths without necessity. As we have seen, some of the most violent reactions have been checked after a reasonable period of scientific sleuthing, treating and prescribing.

Let's stop talking about the next fellow. Let us suppose that tomorrow you develop a rash, not on your arm where your sleeve will cover it, and not on your back where your shirt will conceal its presence. The rash is right on the side of your face, the first thing everyone sees when they come in contact with you. What is your psychological reaction? Will you behold the rash in a mirror, shrug your shoulders and dismiss it from your mind?

That rash becomes your personal problem and, until the problem is solved, your personality suffers.

The first thought is escapism. You don't want to see anyone and you don't want anyone to see you. You soon find that you can't escape reality and that you are only getting in deeper and deeper. The rash is not improving, you're missing time from work and something has to be done.

You ultimately decide that a physician is better able to diagnose your case, so you brace yourself for the ordeal of facing the world while you go to the doctor's office.

You are fortunate that you do not believe in miracles, because the physician isn't able to perform one. All he can do is to start you through his customary medical mill, and explain that you will have to make the best of things until he discovers the source of the rash. Meanwhile, convinced that, whatever it is, it is not contagious, you agree to return to work.

You know the rash is not contagious, and the doctor knows, but does the public know? You will find everybody a bit skeptical about your story, and, although some of your friends and co-workers assure you that they understand, in their own minds they are wondering whether you really have leprosy.

Carrying your brand about with you for a period of time, being stared at by people you don't know, shunned by those you do know—these are the factors that will influence the alteration of your behavior. To make things worse, the rash continues to spread until it covers most of your face, as well as your neck, and other portions of your body not exposed to view.

Several weeks of this, then, perhaps, several months, and you adopt a new doctrine: defeatism. Life has turned against you, has taken away your normal appearance; you have practically forgotten how to laugh; your friendly nature has subsided so that you speak only when unable to avoid doing so, and you terminate your conversations quickly. You have become phlegmatic, and even the sunniest days are cloudy to you, for the brilliant sunshine seems only to mock your anguished condition.

Your interests become limited. Regular club and organization routine disappears from your schedule. Attractions outside your home are practically nil, and you are content to be alone evening after evening, interested primarily in clearing the one hurdle between you and a normal life.

As a result, your transformed psychological outlook, curtailed interests, withdrawal from activity, altered mood and generally subnormal behavior impair the quality of your personality.

The foregoing supposition of what could happen to you is only a portion of the story. You, as an adult, have developed a personality. When the source of the trouble has been found and the trouble itself eradicated, it is quite likely that, within a reasonable length of time, you will drift back to your characteristic manner of projecting yourself.

There is a story of greater basic concern, and it deals with the formative effect of bodily sensitivity upon the personality of youngsters. To see how it works, let us turn to the case of the unluckiest child in the world. This time we shall rear him from the psychological point of view.

Being born with a marked weakness for certain things, he readily yields, and the irritants do their dirty work. The parents, grieved with the thought that their son may be a weakling, are encouraged by the pediatrician's belief that the child will outgrow these sensitivities. Meanwhile, they take all precautions. If a careful diet is necessary, that is what Junior will get.

Growing a bit older, Junior begins to realize that he is getting special care and a lot of attention. By the process of experimentation, he soon discovers that he can have his own way quite easily. At first, his wishes become requests. Later, the requests become demands.

Not wishing to upset the child, the parents capitulate to these demands, giving the child further momentum, and building within him the egoism essential to the development of a "spoiled brat."

As he grows, his desire, both for attention and for his own way about things, is accentuated. He has friends who bow to his whims, but those who refuse to resume pampering where his mother and dad left off are unwelcome in his life.

As time passes, he becomes more and more difficult, expecting everyone to cater to him. Those who do must expect to mold their lives to conform with his. Subconsciously, then, exhibitionism creeps into his personality makeup.

As manhood approaches, his traits begin to fix themselves permanently. With a run of good fortune, he may be able to continue through life, forcing his opinions upon people. On the other hand, he may, and probably will, find many sad disappointments in his life.

Let us view some of the more common forms of sensitivity and the psychological effect they have upon personal behavior.

Basically recognized as one of the most prevalent is "hay fever." Commonly regarded as something terribly funny (when someone else has it), plain, ordinary hay fever is the undoing of hundreds of thousands of personalities each year. Even in its simple stages, it causes weeks of untold discomfort, for it attacks the highly sensitive membranes of the nose.

Only those afflicted are qualified to realize the injustice dealt to sufferers of this bodily reaction, for they alone know the feeling of a nose full of pepper, refusing to respond to hours of blowing. They alone know the agony of a dozen successive sneezes and of red eyes, glassy with tears.

So long as the average hay-fever sufferer does not need to be in bed, and so long as the ailment itself is not contagious, general opinion will continue to classify hay fever as a reaction of the body that is not too serious.

The attitude is totally unfounded, since the effect of this first-class discomfiture upon the projection of one's personality more than offsets its apparent harmlessness as a disease.

During the fall days, when weeds are pollinating and noses running, a dozen large, clean hankies, or a giant-sized box of disposable tissues, supplant the victim's desire for practically anything in the world. He is interested primarily in the relief of his malady.

The necessity of hiding behind a large hanky for nine out of every 10 minutes somehow draws only witty sym-

pathy from those in his company. If the victim is a
gentleman, someone generally takes advantage of the
opportunity to blame hay fever upon the "weeds" under his nose, if he happens to wear a mustache.

Such fun-poking has its ultimate effect upon the vic-
timized individual. He becomes self-conscious and develops the feeling that there is always something wrong
with his face. He is haunted by the constant fear that his
nose or his eyes are running, or that he will sneeze
unexpectedly into the face of a business prospect.

It is to be expected that these fears will eventually
show their effect upon the person's behavior. Very often,
a feeling of inferiority develops. On the other hand, the
person with a nervous disposition may react differently.
He may become disagreeable, grumbling at everything
and everyone.

The effect of "rose fever" is quite similar, except for
the fact that it goes to work earlier in the year, when the
grass and trees begin to pollinate.

Either hay fever or "rose fever" permitted to gnaw
into one's body for a long period of time often makes
way for a good case of asthma. Here, of course, the
friendly joking comes to an end, for, although a nice,
long wheeze may have the sound of a tin whistle, everyone realizes that such wheezing makes breathing very
difficult.

Asthma, too, has its psychological difficulties. Those
afflicted subsconsciously cultivate the habit of apolo-
gizing for their asthmatic attacks. This is a defense
mechanism, used because the victims fear what others
may be thinking about them.

And how about the individual who simply cannot
get along with strawberries? At the strawberry festival,
he eats heartily, and almost promptly breaks out in a
blushing rash which keeps everybody away from him,

believing that whatever he has may be contagious. This is no cheerful thought for the physically sensitive person.

One of the most common words in any language is "headache." Almost everything, from a blonde to a race horse, has, at one time or another, been accused of causing headaches. Considerable research has come to place a good deal of the responsibility for them upon bodily sensitivity.

The kind of headache a man gets from a blonde is purely mental. We are concerned primarily with headaches that hurt. Aside from such obvious causes as sinus infection, strained eyes, a cold in the head, an upset stomach or a hangover, headaches may often come from a thing as simple as a codfish ball or an apricot.

Regardless of what the irritant is that is causing your headache, you are generally very poor company when you have one. And, if you complain perennially about it, you will soon find yourself a very unpopular person. This constant pain in the cerebral region definitely affects your personality as it is projected to those about you. Can you expect to register dynamically? Not unless you're a good enough actor to conceal your feelings, and few of use are.

The solution to a problem in sensitivity may seem to be a simple one. In many instances it is. A restricted diet, cautiously observed, is often the most effective means of avoiding recurrences of the difficulty, whatever it may be. A series of treatments by a competent physician will often build one's resistance to the irritant that has been making him ill.

The story does not end here. The cases demanding far greater sacrifices are legion. In plain words, this business of unusual or altered reaction is often more serious than it appears on the surface. It takes little character to eliminate garlic from the diet, but it takes great courage to make a major adjustment in your manner of living.

Can you place yourself in the position of the man who, after being a baker all his life, learned that the only way to preserve his health was to change jobs?

Perhaps you are now working at a trade you have spent years learning. Suddenly you take ill and the doctor tells you to give up your job. You'll have to start all over and learn something new, simply because your body reacts negatively toward printing ink, wheat, silk or fur.

As a furrier with years of experience, you suddenly find yourself faced with a serious problem. There is no branch of the business where furs are not handled to some extent. Where are you to turn? What are you to do?

A degree more serious, and of greater effect upon the personality and mental attitude of a person, is the realization that a particular sensitivity will only be checked by removal to a different climate. Consider the sacrifices that must be made: change of work or transfer to a new and foreign branch; complete disruption of social life; breaking up of the home; transferring of children to new and unfamiliar schools and, in general, a new start in life.

It must not be reasoned that only the individuals afflicted with such supersensitivity are affected. A man whose body refuses to accept orris root in any of its forms can make life pretty sad and uninteresting for his wife. Likewise, she can make things pretty uncomfortable for him, if she refuses to cooperate. In such as case, cooperation would involve the elimination of certain cosmetics from her feminine routine, for the majority of cosmetics contain orris root, an especially irritating substance. The cosmetic market is now covered for such emergencies, of course, by the evolution of products that do not contain this irritant.

Many cases on record have demonstrated that the presence of an irritant on either husband or wife was nearly responsible for marital disunion. One in particular comes to mind, concerning a young couple married less than a year.

They approached an attorney and spoke to him of "incompatibility." During the course of the interview, when the woman was asked to justify her charges, she innocently explained that, during their brief wedded life, her husband had rarely been able to perform his marital duties.

The husband told the attorney that he was subject to serious asthmatic attacks, and that such attacks invariably came at the wrong time.

A physician friend of the attorney saw more truth than humor in the husband's plight. With some effort, he secured permission to examine the husband. His theory proved to be right. The husband, sensitive to orris root, was merely reacting to the large quantities of it contained in a scented dusting powder his wife used on her body after bathing.

Not thoroughly convinced that the couple was beyond the point of reconciliation, the attorney, upon the recommendation of the doctor, asked that the wife discontinue the use of any dusting powders, and make another attempt to get along with her husband.

Much to the gratification of the couple, and to the satisfaction of the attorney, the case never got to the courthouse.

Another situation with the incompatibility angle concerned a man who had taken about all he could stand from his wife. With them, life was one merry battle after another. The wife was irritable to the point at which even the slightest slip of the tongue would cause her to have a tantrum. The husband felt more and more henpecked until, one day, he decided that he would take matters into his own hands.

His attorney advised that perhaps the wife was ill. A chronic ailment might easily have been the cause of her excitability. Reflecting, the husband recalled that his wife had been complaining about insomnia. It seemed as though they had hardly gotten to bed when she began coughing and wheezing. A physician properly diagnosed her difficulty as asthma, but seemed unable to locate the specific contributing factor. After a number of weeks of unsuccessful questioning, the woman broke down and offered vital information which she had previously withheld because of its personal nature.

Her husband perspired freely, and had developed a phobia, a morbid fear, of B.O. Inasmuch as his work brought him constantly in contact with people, he took precautions against this body odor by practically covering his body with strongly scented dusting powder after each bath.

It was this dusting powder that was primarily responsible for the wife's asthma, hence her insomnia and her irritable, disagreeable attitude which nearly brought destruction to their married life.

One of the most interesting cases, in which a double sensitivity for the same irritant was nearly responsible for the ruin of two lives, concerned a young couple who had gone to see their attorneys regarding divorce. Each of them claimed there was infidelity on the part of the other, for they had both developed a nasty rash about their genital organs. Each sadly confessed to his attorney that the other was responsible for a venereal disease recently contracted.

"Are you certain that's what you have?" one of the attorneys asked.

"Well, not exactly. But what else could it be?" replied the man.

"Have you been to see a physician?"

"No."

"Why don't you do that instead of trying to diagnose your own case?"

Individually, the couple went for medical examinations. Individually, they learned that what they had was not a venereal disease but merely a sensitivity to one of the ingredients in a new contraceptive jelly they had begun to use. When the medical reports were given to the two attorneys, they were convinced that infidelity was not the case at all. The clients were brought in and both husband and wife convinced each other that a serious mistake had been made, and that reconciliation was the only logical move.

Still another kind of psychological reaction to sensitivity concerns the family that is emotionally upset over the poor health of children. The father may earn a very meager wage, most of which is absorbed by the necessities of rent, food, clothing and utilities. Little is left for luxuries, and practically nothing is left for doctor bills.

Disaster strikes the household, and for months the doctor gets most of the income. The family morale drops to a new low each day, and life seems futile. Week after week, the family debt grows while the scant income continues at its low ebb.

This constant pressure lowers the personality projection level of the entire family, until each member comes to face the world as a beaten, sordid bit of humanity.

Large sums of money had been wasted in a hit-or-miss method of trying to find out what is wrong with the child or children. It isn't until the difficulty is traced to a certain dust on the father's clothing, carried home from the factory, that real progress is made with the case. By this time, the damage is done, and even the recovery of the child is unable to raise the family morale to the position it held prior to the illness.

Distressing, indeed, is a frustrated romance. Although two individuals have professed their love for each other, the girl refuses to chain her sweetheart to a lifelong invalid. She is abnormally underweight and cannot seem to gain, regardless of the fact that she takes halibut liver oil capsules and gets all the food and rest prescribed by the family doctor.

The young lady, afflicted with a perpetual cold, has decided that she has tuberculosis.

Their young love thwarted, each did all in his power to forget. Later the boy met another—not quite the same—and she made him a good wife. But the first love was never dead, for he carried it about in a tiny corner of his heart.

It was not until a number of years later that the girl, persuaded to be tested for sensitivities, learned that the halibut oil she had been taking all those years was a poison her body could not fight off. It was this which had kept her from gaining weight, and which kept her in the perpetual state of apparently having a cold. Having eliminated the fish liver oil from her diet, she soon built herself to a state of health she had never dared dream she would achieve. But the greater wound was still there; her love was gone.

What is to be learned from all this? We can reasonably be certain that the arm of possibility is far-reaching where sensitivities are concerned, and that their effect upon the projected personality of an individual is equally as prominent as, and ultimately of greater concern than, the physical manifestation.

We learn that, in the course of living, we are constantly offering our personalities for sale, in one way or another, and that anything which scathes the presentation of these personalities must be considered an enemy, to be eliminated as quickly as possible.

In our discussion we were concerned with how the patient is influenced by his allergy. I am certain that you, the reader, are interested in the *why* of these psychosomatic reactions. With authorities on the subject it is claimed that the psyche (mind) is disturbed for some unconscious reason, uses an organ (the nose, lungs or skin) as a "voice" to express its disturbance, and in the process, produces an allergic disease such as asthma, hay fever or hives. Unresolved conflicts, arrested development and fixations as discussed by Freud result in immature behavior and unrealistic attempts at resolving problems, which in turn result in excessive physical activity of an organ, and that in its turn may result in—say—asthma. Such a response is claimed to be a suppressed cry of an individual, separated or threatened by separation from the mother figure.

Such psychological concepts are, however, not generally accepted as an explanation of allergic disease. It is important, however, to recognize that the body has a mind, and often a specialist in allergy and one in psychiatry can work together for mutual benefit in restoring a patient's health both allergically and emotionally.

It must be acknowledged that there are parents who overwhelm their children; they seem to engulf them and overprotect them, "smothering" them. This is due to fear, guilt or frustration, for many reasons which cannot be gone into in this book. However, the effect on all members of the immediate family and other relatives makes it important to understand that there are strong emotional factors present in allergy, as in other chronic illnesses, and they must be dealt with. We must state that our own experience has yet not revealed a single case of allergy due purely to the emotions, though they may be very strong in a given patient. There is no doubt, however, that strong emotions can aggravate the allergy.

Let us consider Bobby T., an eight-year-old boy, who lived in a hostile enviornment. The parents were always fighting—verbally, at any rate. Bobby frequently had attacks of wheezing with shortness of breath and coughing, "colds" with sore throat and fever often as high as 104 degrees. Each of his parents treated him with great care and he was brought in regularly for treatment, but we were able to give him little relief with our usually successful allergy management and care. We recommended sending him to an institution for severe asthmatic children, away from his environment, and specially away from his parents ("Parentectomy" —removal of parents). Within 24 hours after he was admitted he stopped wheezing and became free from his other symptoms as well. For one year he was seen frequently by one of us (JAR). He played actively and lost no schooling. During this period his parents were divorced. When the boy returned home, his parents could no longer create the old insecurity in him. He then responded successfully to allergic care and treatment.

CHAPTER

22 Complications Resulting from Neglect of Allergy

IF YOU have ever been the victim of a habitual back-slapper or cheek-pincher, you have undoubtedly felt the distressing sensation of being pinched or slapped on precisely the same spot each time. Each attack upon your cheek or your back feels just so much worse than the last one, until, eventually, a painful swelling or a black-and-blue mark appears.

Assuming, for our purpose, that the human body is analogous to an electric circuit, the swelling or the black-and-blue mark is the point at which you "blew a fuse." Being the least resistant point in an electrical circuit, the fuse is the point where the trouble comes to a head.

Figuratively speaking, the human body is also protected by fuses. These are the points of least resistance within the body, and they naturally differ with the individual.

The attacks which eventually cause you to "blow a fuse" need not come from without. We have learned that a "short circuit" within the body itself is very often the source of the difficulty.

Each and every one of thousands and thousands of irritants known to affect our bodies has its own way of finding one of our weaknesses, and of working on it until it becomes scarred in one way or another.

But here is where we differ from the electrical circuit, for, when a fuse is blown, the trouble is automatically checked. The same cannot be said about the human body. Any irritant is capable of producing a chronic maladjustment in any part of the body. Left unchecked, these irritants will gnaw viciously at the body until the damage is almost beyond repair.

But this is not all. When corn, clams or cranberries take a dislike to your body, their abuse affects the whole structure, even though the mucous membranes of the nasal passage or the cartilage of the hip joint bear the brunt of the attacks.

Generally speaking, sensitivity to any irritant often affects your height, weight or the condition of your blood composition. It may easily alter your nervous or digestive systems, making you an excitable, high-strung individual, whose food does not digest completely. You may have a run-down feeling, with low blood pressure and low metabolism.

These are facts. They are not intended to terrorize you. As facts, they do not concern us nearly so much as the ultimate complications to which they may lead. A body weakened by some irritant becomes vulnerable to attacks of really serious illnesses.

What happens to the child afflicted for the first five or six years of his life with a sensitive breathing condition? The abnormal breathing conditions cause him to distort his face and develop a receding chin somewhat reminiscent of the comic character, Andy Gump. A receding lower jaw, together with flattened cheekbones, add to the improper development of the head. Perennial nasal conditions eventually block the sinus passages, causing sinus infection.

We must not overlook the fact that the improper development of the head is the greatest source of poorly formed, poorly focused eyes and crooked teeth. The nasal connection with the ear canals controls our sense of balance.

Often an adult who consults a physician with regard to difficulty in breathing is told that there is a small "bone" that must be removed from the nose. Although these small "bones" are often removed, they return because the basic difficulty—elimination of the irritant causing them—is not effected.

Moving downward to the chest cavity, we find that fuses blown in this portion of the body often take the form of chronic hoarseness, bronchitis or even bronchial abscess. Very often, these are accompanied by bad breath and a disagreeable odor from the mouth.

Such difficulty in getting air into the lungs must be compensated for, so the lungs become overdeveloped. To accommodate these enlarged organs, more room is needed and a barrel-shaped chest results, generally giving the appearnce of top-heaviness.

Then, too, there is the heart to be considered. An excess strain put on any part of the body is felt by the heart. Such strain as the lungs undergo during asthmatic or bronchial breathing will cause the heart to overdevelop in order to accommodate the strain. The overdevelopment is often responsible for chronic heart conditions.

But, should the sensitivity take the low road and strike through the gastrointestinal tract, we can be fairly certain that there will be stomach irritations and chronic heartburn, more alarmingly described in TV commercials as gastric hyperacidity. This is ultimately responsible for stomach ulcers, bowel irritation, constipation or hemorrhoids.

Attacking our basic structure, an irritant or group of irritants sometimes makes a fuse of our bones. This comes in the form of calcium deficiency, and, unless you have been able to escape reading dairy advertisements, you'll readily understand that lack of this mineral in the bones makes them soft and brittle.

We come, finally, to the open-air theater of sensitivity: the skin rash, in all its forms, that turns eventually to a more serious, and often distasteful, case of eczema.

There is the case of Joseph D., who, after suffering from chronic asthma during the greater part of his 58 years, visited the doctor and learned that he would have done well to care for a heart condition during the past five years.

Diagnosis proved that the latter condition was obviously a result of a sensitivity to walnuts. But, before an all-out course of treatment could be prescribed to cure the asthma, the heart condition had to be relieved. Once this was done, the problem of walnuts once more took on importance, and, after a year's treatment, not only the heart condition, but the asthma as well, was eliminated.

Highly interesting, from the standpoint of what can actually be done, is the case of Dorothy A., whose undernourished, underweight, anemic, asthmatic condition was enough to frighten the physician when she entered his office.

Yes, hay fever—simple, old hay fever—was her difficulty. Start a full scale series of hay fever treatments? No. Dorothy was only advised to avoid pollen, but, at the same time, she took shots of liver extract and treatments designed to build her up physically into a normal individual, after which the counterattack on ragweed pollen was carried out with easy success

How would you feel if you had spent nearly five years of your life unable to speak in little more than a whisper? This happened to Fred Y., who was also quite run down at the time he was referred to the physician for sensitivity examination.

Preliminary questioning placed him unequivocally in the ranks of constipated individuals. The same dfficulty that had blown out the basement fuse went to work on the second floor, and, before long, his normal voice had become hoarse, then the hoarse voice succumbed to the whisper.

The doctor's obvious task was first to clear up Fred's physical condition, which he did, at the same time keeping the patient on a very strict diet. Gradually the voice returned, as the constipation cleared.

CHAPTER

23 *Treatment of Allergy*

Injection Treatment of Allergy

WHEN COMPLETE avoidance of allergens is impossible or impractical, hyposensitization of injectons with inhalants including pollens should be employed. Since there remains a group of inhalant-sensitive patients who react to a minimal exposure, injection treatment becomes a necessity. Almost all of these patients receive good relief by hyposensitization injections of extracts of the inhalant substances to which they are allergic. The extract material in various dilutions may be obtained from several reliable laboratories. The materials are mixtures of the environmental inhalant allergens. The dose schedule depends on the experience of the physician allergist, the environment and the patient's sensitivity. The principle is to begin treatments with varied diluted subcutaneous injections gradually increasing the dose until a concentration is reached, at which time the patient states that he is relieved. The practice of giving these injections depends on the experience of the allergist. Some give doses as high as the patient will tolerate and others give varied dilute concentrations. We believe giving the right concentration depends on the patient's total response to the treatment. When the relief is obtained the schedule having begun at twice weekly intervals is gradually reduced to weekly intervals, bi-monthly and monthly intervals. This will vary again according to the patient's needs. The treatment continues over a period of some years. In our experience it is wise to maintain the injections at three or four weekly intervals indefinitely.

"One Shot" injection treatment was devised for the purpose of reducing the number and frequency of hyposensitizing injections. The method as it is being given today needs to be improved. Tests for determining degree of sensitivity are cumbersome. Severe reactions are encountered; abcesses and lumps at the site of injections have been reported, and that they remain for long periods. What happens to the oil emulsion which is injected? These and other questions must be answered before the method can be used generally. Men and women of excellent scientific abilities, either laud or condemn the method. We feel that it can be used with great caution in very selective instances. Great skill is, however, needed to make this determination.

The latest injection treatment is a preparation in which the allergic substances are precipitated by a special chemical known as Pyridine. The Pyridine complex is used with alum and the final material can then be redissolved in a salt solution. The treatments are given by injection in exactly the same manner as the regular treatments. The advantages are fewer injections and apparently a high degree of safety. This treatment is still under investigation.

Drug Treatment in Allergy

Drugs commonly used in allergy are known to most sufferers with allergic conditions. If they are correctly used, they can provide the greatest benefit.

Antihistamines: There are nearly 100 different preparations available. Nearly all have side effects, such as drowsiness, dizziness and, in some cases, nausea and vomiting. They are, however, if carefully chosen, of great value in hay fever and in some cases of hives, small or large. They are of some value in itching of the skin. Few other allergic conditions are relieved, and no allergy is cured by them.

Research investigators of the antihistamines have demonstrated that most antihistamines fall into four distinct chemical groups, each group having somewhat different action. They are variously named by the different drug manufacturing companies into a great many products. Some are combined with other drugs which are supposed to enhance the effect of the antihistamine. The following are representative important examples:

Group 1.   Benedryl (Park Davis Co.) ; Hydryllin (G. D. Searle) ; Dramamine (G. D. Searle) ; Decapryn (Wm. J. Merrell)

Group 2.   Neoantergan (Merck) ; Tagathen (Lederle) ; Thenylene (Abbott) ; Desoxyn (Abbott) ; Hystadyl (Eli Lilly) ; Thenfadil (Winthrop) ; Phenergan (Wyeth)

Group 3.   Chlortrimeton (Schering) ; Coricidin (Schering) ; Pyronil (Eli Lilly) ; CoPyronil (Eli Lilly) ; Orinade Spansules (Smith, Kline & French)

Group 4.   Antistine (Ciba) ; Perazil (Burrows & Welcome) ; Actidil (B. & W.) ; Actified (B. & W.) ; Thephorin (Roche) ; Dimetane (A. H. Robbins) ; Dimetapp (A. H. Robbins)

Antibiotics: The discovery of the sulfa drugs, penicillin and the others which followed, has made a great impact on medicine and upon allergy, in particular. Infection in asthma will usually aggravate it and cause recurring severe attacks. With the proper antibiotic in adequate dosage, the infection is quickly controlled. As in all things, there are both good and bad with the antibiotics. Allergic reactions to the sulfa drugs, penicillin and others, can occur when individuals become sensitized to them. A number of antibiotics may certainly be prescribed and their effects carefully observed by your physician. The following are important and are used for specific reasons: Gantrisin (Roche) ; Kynex (Lederle) ; Terramycin and Aureomycin, produced by nearly all large drug manufacturers and distributors under varying names. Achromycin (Lederle) ; Erythromycin (Abbott) ; Lincocin (Upjohn) ; Loridin (Eli Lilly) ; Keflex (Eli Lilly) ; Vibramycin (Pfizer) ; Panmycin (Upjohn) ; Macrodantin and Furidantin (Eaton Laboratories) ; Mycostatin (Squibb) ; Minocin (Lederle) ; and TAO (Roerig).

Bronchodilators: These are antispasmodic drugs, and are used to relax the muscle spasm of the bronchial tubes in the asthmatic individual. They also reduce the swelling of the mucous membranes, thereby allowing the phlegm to be brought up with ease. The two most commonly used drugs are adrenalin and ephedrine. Adrenalin is given either by injection or spray. The solutions are of different concentration and should be prescribed by a physician. Ephedrine is the oral preparation used similarly, but not as effectively. Ephedrine has been combined with aminophyllin and phenobarbitol, and, in some cases, is more effective. There are many preparations available with adrenalin or ephedrine, and they act in much the same way.

The basis for most of the preparations used in this category are derived from the action of the epinephrine or ephedrine base. Some drug manufacturers have added medications which they believe prolongs their effects. A few of the bronchodilators available are: Bronkephrine Hydrochloride Aerosol (George Breon);

Bronkotabs (G. Breon) ; Duohaler (Riker) ; Duomedi-
haler (Riker) ; Duovent (Riker) ; Isuprel, Mistometer,
(Winthrop) ; Norisodrine Aerohaler (Abbott); Vapo-
nephrin (USV Pharmeceutical) ; Vapo-N-Iso (USV
Pharmeceutical) ; Marax (Roerig) ; Tedral (Warner-
Chilcott) ; Sus-phrine (Cooper) ; Ephedrine Sulphate
(Eli Lilly) . All the above are aerosos.

Dermatology Preparations: These must be chosen on
the basis of sound medical principles. For the extremely
acute, so-called "red hot," swollen, blistered, oozing
skin rash, baths, packs, wet dressings and anti-infective
substances of a non-greasy nature may be used. When
drying has resulted and scales are present, shake lotions
may be used. For older or chronic skin rashes, stronger
stimulating and healing ointments may be used.

Nearly all drug firms have special skin preparations
for the treatment of allergy of the skin. They all contain cortisone in varying strengths, and are creams,
ointments or suspensions. Some preparations are: Ceta-
cort (Texas Pharmical) ; Cort Dome Creme & Lotion
(Dome) ; Kenalog Creme, Lotion, Ointment or Spray
(Squibbs) ; Syntex Creme and Lotion (Syntex) ; Vali-
sone (Schering) ; Vioform-Hydrocortisone (Ciba) ;
Decadron (Merck, Sharpe & Dome) .

Hormones: Adrenal gland hormones used for the
relief of the allergies are technically known as adreno-
cortical hormones, and are produced in the cortex of
the adrenal gland, which sits on top of the kidneys.
This substance is produced either directly or by a hor-
mone in the anterior part of the pituitary gland, which
is at the base of the brain. The substance first discovered
was known as cortisone. However, further study and
research has found more potent hormones which give

equal or greater relief with smaller doses and fewer side effects; they are hydrocortisone, prednisone, prednisolone, dexamethasone, betamethasone and others. These steroids should not be taken unless a physician experienced in their harmful effects keeps a careful eye on the patient. Too much, too little, stopping them too soon and not observing the rules of salt and water retention will result in swellings, retention of sodium, depletion of potassium, disturbance of the protein metabolism, with reversal of nitrogen balance, and interference with sugar metabolism and storage, with resulting increase in blood sugar and the presence of sugar in the urine.

There is an increase in acid in the stomach, along with pepsin, and possible production of ulcers of the stomach. The nervous system can be seriously involved, causing serious depression, changes of mood and, at times, actual mental change. There are many other possible side effects, including an increase in blood pressure, interference in the healing of wounds and some superimposed infections.

When such untoward effects result, the physician must be there to treat them promptly, with the necessary medicines to overcome the swellings, with diuretics, with insulin to reduce the sugar and the antibiotics for the intercurrent infection. These are potent drugs and should only be used with great care.

Sedatives, Hypnotics and Tranquilizers: This group of drugs can be of great benefit to relieve pain, itching and burning, and, thereby, afford the individual rest and sleep. The following should certainly not be taken on one's own initiative, but on recommendation by his physician or allergist. Among those frequently recommended are: Valium (Roche); Librium (Roche);

Delmane (Roche) ; Equanil (Wyeth) ; Doriden (USV Pharmaceutical) ; Placidyl (Abbott) or Miltown (Wallace) (McKesson & Robbins). These drugs are similar but vary in intensity. When used for quieting effect, they are sedatives; when used in larger doses and at night, they are called hypnotics, producing sleep. Tranquilizers are used for producing the mildest sedation. This term has become quite popular.

All drugs in this category have themselves produced allergies. The use of drugs in any of these groups should not be taken lightly, although they can be of much benefit properly used. They can also be habit-forming and sensitizing.

Aminophyllin: Aminophyllin is a well-known drug to most individuals who have bronchial asthma. It has been administered by mouth, into the muscle or vein by injection and has been given by rectum in liquid or suppository form. Relief has been good in some instances. The main problem when taken by mouth has been the inability of the patient to take a large enough dose to give adequate benefit, due to the irritating effect on the stomach. It may cause nausea or vomiting in some cases and must therefore be discontinued.

In recent years, preparations have been manufactured to overcome this complication: Choledyl, Cardalin and Theo-Nar are oral preparations which we have used. In our experience, we have found Theo-Nar to be effective for relief, without any observed untoward reactions on the stomach or otherwise.

There are many combinations which will assist in dilating the bronchial tubes, reduce the swelling of the mucous membrane, and assist in thinning the mucus which will be expectorated more easily and relieve the patient. To mention a few, they are: Elixophyllin and

Elixophyllin K I (Cooper); Lufyllin preparations (Mallinckrodt); Quibron (Mead Johnson); Verequad (Knoll); Fleet Theophyllin (Fleet); and many others.

In recent years they have been researching various drugs, but only one in England appears to be effective in fairly extensive trials with asthmatic adults and children. It has not yet been approved by the Federal Drug Agency (FDA) in the U.S. The chemical name is disodium cromoglycate; it will no doubt have a company name when it becomes available, which should be soon. It has proven to be an effective drug for the relief of wheezing and in causing an improvement in general physical well being; it makes possible a reduction in the number of other drugs required, including the various cortisone preparations. It appears to have definite protective action against bronchospasm (tightening of the muscles of the bronchial tubes, which causes shortness of breath and wheezing sounds) in the lungs.

There are also mechanical methods of delivering epinephrine and other bronchodilators in combination with physiological salt solution, alcohol, and preparations to thin the secretions in the bronchial tubes. The Benett and Bird machine's intermittent positive pressure action assists in breathing as well. With instructions from your doctor they can be used at home. Other machines will deliver straight oxygen; still others fine vapor moisture, but they are subject to close and careful observation as in some instances they may be ineffective or cause some difficulty in the condition.

Vitamins: Vitamins, especially B and ascorbic acid, are found to protect cells and have a beneficial effect on the very important adrenal gland. Multiple vitamins contain the essential ones and are of great value to allergic individuals when they are on very limited diets. There are many known essential vitamins; these can be found in most retail drug and food establishments everywhere.

Note Well: Barbiturates and the derivatives of opium can be very harmful for asthmatics and there are quite a number of fatalities reported from their use. Aside from becoming allogenic, they effect the entire respiratory breathing mechanism adversely in the asthmatic.

Climate in Allergy

This should not be taken too lightly, for one must consider the transplanting of an entire family, with economic, sociologic and psychologic implications. The following guides may be important for anyone contemplating such a change.

It is wise first to consider a trial temporary change for three to six months. If certain allergens, such as pollen, are known factors in one climatic location, and this has been confirmed by allergic study, a change to a climate not containing such substances may be tried. When infection has been a recurring factor, a change to a climate where the incidence of infection is much less may be advisable. The change to a hot, dry or hot, humid climate depends on the existing allergy. A change may remove a psychological barrier and be helpful.

Hypnosis and Allergy

When allergic symptoms are present but personality abberations due to psychogenic alterations exist, it is obvious that the disturbed personality requires the primary treatment. In such cases, it becomes most important to treat the total patient, including the personality as well as the body.

Certain allergies can be cured by hypnosis. It is of greatest importance if hypnosis is used that it be accomplished by a physician who understands the effects on the mind and body of the patient. Hypnosis can be very dangerous if it is carried out by one unskilled in medicine and psychiatry. It may aggravate the entire problem and even result in a complete mental breakdown.

There are three components responsible for the severity of an allergy. These are the allergic, physical and psychogenic factors. The allergenic component has been described with a number of case illustrations. The physical component includes any abnormality in body function, regardless of the cause. This will retard improvement of an allergy unless it is corrected. Finally, the psychogenic component is the most difficult to evaluate, as it may be either apparent or hidden from conscious thought. When the cause is apparent and the individual does not have the ability to overcome it, hypnotic therapy can be of help in carefully selected patients. When the underlying difficulty is deep-seated in the subconscious, regression under a skillful medical hypnotist may bring it to the conscious level, where the patient can recognize and deal with it intelligently. Let us again emphasize, however, that each individual with allergy must be carefully evaluated before hypnosis is attempted. No harm will result from the use of this technique by one aware of the medical problems involved.

CHAPTER

24 Do-It-Yourself Procedures for the Allergies

IN THE TREATMENT of allergic symptoms, many procedures are employed. They are aids, for the most part, in removing allergens from the environment and the diet. We believe we have stressed sufficiently the need for a full study of the allergic, physical and psychosomatic factors and the need for specific treatment directed at overcoming the abnormal ones.

The following pages are devoted to implementing and assisting in the removal of allergens, and are stated, for the most part, in outline form. It is to be remembered that, although one allergen, such as milk, dust or egg, may have initiated the allergy, the absence of study and care in the early stages has permitted the condition to become complicated. Additional allergens and factors of body and mind have added to the distress. The avoidance of the original allergen will not control the allergy at this stage. All physical and emotional factors must be corrected, and the secondary contributing allergens must be eliminated. It can, therefore, be seen that the earlier an allergy is treated the better.

Allergic management is essential to accomplish relief of distress and prevention of complications, which may be very serious. Elimination of the most common allergens in major foods is outlined. Recipes and substitute foods are prescribed to assist the allergic individual and to enable him to maintain a normal existence.

Recommended Prophylactic Measures for Expectant Mothers in Allergic Families*

1. Every effort should be made to breast-feed the baby as completely as possible. We know that the completely breast-fed infant has seven times as many chances of escaping eczema as the bottle-fed baby.

2. The mother should eat no eggs during her pregnancy. This does not mean that she should be on an egg-free diet, but eggs as such and foods consisting largely of eggs, such as angel cakes or custard, should be avoided.

3. She should not drink an excessive amount of cow's milk. A pint a day should be given, preferably boiled 10 minutes, but, in addition to this, calcium and phosphorus should be supplied in adequate quantities from other sources, as, for example, two or three times a day. Cheese, except in minimal amounts, is also to be avoided.

4. The mother who is herself allergic should avoid those foods and other allergens which, she knows, cause her trouble.

5. She should eat a rather wide variety of food and not concentrate, as pregnant women occasionally do, on just a few articles of diet.

6. The above directions should be followed as long as the baby is nursed. When the mother stops nursing the baby, she may return to the diet she was on before pregnancy.

Prevention of Allergic Diseases in Your New Baby*

Most people know that the tendency to suffer from allergic diseases runs in families, *i.e.*, is inherited. Doctors regard the prevention of disease, which is called

* From the office of Jerome Glaser, M.D., Rochester, N.Y. and with his permission. (modified)

prophylaxis, as the most important way to treat a disease. Studies in Rochester, carried out by us for a period of more than 20 years, indicate that, if you or your husband or any of your children suffer from an allergic disease, the chances are that the new baby in your family, whom we call "a potentially allergic infant," will, in 60 per cent of cases (six out of every 10), develop a major allergic disease, such as eczema, hay fever, asthma or allergic rhinitis (also called "chronic catarrh," chronic "sinus" or "one cold after another"), before the age of six years.

Our studies indicate that proper management of the mother during pregnancy, and, particularly, of the newborn baby will reduce the infant's chances of acquiring a major allergic disease before the age of six years from 60 per cent to 15 per cent. In other words, your child will have almost as good a chance of escaping allergic disease as if there were no allergy in your family. Since the procedures advocated are simple and harmless in the hands of well-trained physicians, it is very much worthwhile to make the attempt.

During pregnancy, the mother is given a special diet, because there is some evidence that the unborn child may be sensitized by foods ingested by the mother. These foods are particularly milk and eggs, so the diet is low in milk and omits egg. The proteins of the diet are made up by meats and the minerals by special preparations. Because almost anything the mother eats or drinks during nursing may pass through to the child in the breast milk, the mother should remain on this diet throughout the period she nurses the baby.

It is highly important for the mother to nurse the baby because, as we have said, the breast-fed infant has seven times as many chances of escaping eczema as does the bottle-fed baby, and over 80 per cent of the infants with eczema go on to develop the other important allergic diseases listed earlier.

If the mother cannot or will not nurse the baby or, for some reason, the breast-feeding must be stopped, then the infant should be fed soybean milk immediately, with no cow's milk feedings whatsoever from birth, or at any other time, until the age of six to nine months, when the infant may, in the great majority of cases, be changed to cow's milk without difficulty. It is somewhat more difficult to get a baby started on soybean milk than on cow's milk, but this can be done successfully in over 85 per cent of cases.

IF YOU WOULD LIKE TO FOLLOW THIS METHOD OF ATTEMPTING TO PREVENT YOUR CHILD FROM DEVELOPING AN ALLERGIC DISEASE, PLEASE BE SURE TO OBTAIN THE APPROVAL OF BOTH YOUR OBSTETRICIAN AND THE PHYSICIAN WHO IS TO TAKE CARE OF THE BABY AFTERWARD.

Prevention of Allergy—General Instructions

1. Keep away from dust. Do not sweep, but, if you must, protect yourself by covering your mouth and nose with several layers of damp gauze.

2. Avoid the use of insect powders in your home; this includes fly sprays, roach and ant powders, dog flea powders and mothproofing preparations. Avoid contact with irritating odors from stoves, lamps, paints, tobacco smoke, camphor and tar.

3. Do not keep pets unless tested specifically for them.

4. Dust precautions are to followed explicitly.

5. Do not overeat. Avoid late evening meals. Avoid carbonated waters such as ginger ale, which forms gas in the stomach.

6. Drink eight glasses of water daily.

7. Exercise moderately by walking. Walk slowly; do not get short of breath by rushing and stopping occasionally.

8. Protect yourself against overexposure to inclement weather so that you do not catch cold.

9. Do not use mustard plasters or flaxseed poultices.

10. Do not take medication unless you have first consulted your doctor about it.

11. Avoid perfumes, face powders, sachets and scented talcum powders, shampoos, toilet water and scented soaps. Many of these contain ingredients which are irritating and cause symptoms.

12. Avoid all dusty and musty places, such as storerooms, closets and so forth.

13. Avoid the foods in the manner recommended on the skin test record obtained by your physician.

14. Avoid swimming unless specifically recommended.

15. Use no condiments, spices, peppers, sauces, mustard, pickles or any other highly seasoned foods like chili.

16. Report for treatments as directed. A condition which has been present for years cannot be eradicated without some patience, effort and cooperation. Do not allow an improvement in this persistent allergic condition to lessen in any way your attention to the above important facts.

Prevention Treatment of Nasal and Bronchial Allergy*

The most important treatment of any disease is prevention. As you know from the study made to determine the cause of the allergy, treatment for the cause

---

* From the office of Jerome Glaser, M.D., Rochester, N.Y., and with his permission.

is carried on for the purpose of ultimate possible cure. Before this can be obtained, however, it is important to prevent acute attacks while the prolonged treatment is going on.

One of the most common causes of the acute attacks of nasal and bronchial allergy at any age is an acute upper respiratory infection. Because of this fact, some believe that infection is the principal cause of this allergy. Because the sufferer from upper or lower respiratory allergy has chronic swelling of the lining membranes and, thus, has poor circulation, he is more subject to allergic attacks when these membranes become infected. The prevention and treatment of these infections is important, but should not relieve one of the necessity for avoiding the basic causes. In some cases, what appears to be the onset of an acute upper respiratory infection may be the expression of an allergic reaction and in no way be related to an infectious agent.

If the upper respiratory infection or "cold" can be prevented, the nasal or asthmatic attack may be prevented. The following suggestions are, therefore, recommended, *with the consent of the family physician.*

1. At the earliest sign of a "cold," immediately begin taking antihistamines. The familiar feeling of general aching, accompanied by a scratchy sensation in the throat and a running nose, is well known.

2. If symptoms continue after 48 hours, administer an antibiotic or anti-infective and follow the instructions on the prescription.

If, in spite of the above measures, the upper respiratory infection progresses and an attack is beginning, the following approach in treatment is recommended.

3. Bed rest is now advised, as it protects from aggra-

vating factors, such as exercise and changes in temperature and humidity.

4. Now begin taking an expectorant cough mixture every three or four hours. This will help loosen the phlegm and enable it to come up more easily; thus attacks will be prevented.

5. Start taking nose drops. Nasal sprays are superior. No oily drops should be used. The drops are best instilled just before meals and during the night, as necessary, to permit nasal breathing.

6. Fluids should be given as much as will be tolerated, and the bowels must be kept freely moving.

7. Steam inhalations may be used when they have been found beneficial in the past.

8. Special allergy tablets (ephedrine, aminophyllin or cortisone) may be taken, if it is believed necessary at this time.

9. Insert an aminophyllin suppository or inject liquid. This should be done nightly until danger of attacks are past.

10. Inhalations or injections of adrenalin will be recommended by your doctor, if indicated as necessary.

Instructions for Physical Exercises to Combat Asthma

Place: In front of open window.

Time: 1. In the morning before breakfast, when you are feeling fresh and are least likely to be asthmatic.

2. At night, before getting into bed, to clear the lungs before sleep.

3. When asthma is coming on; many patients are able to shorten their attacks entirely by doing these simple exercises gently.

Essential Points:

1. Before commencing the exercise, you should blow on a handkerchief to ensure a clear airway.

2. As the object of the exercise is to empty the lungs, each exercise should begin with a short sniff through the nose, followed by a long breath out through the mouth. A whistling noise should be made with the lips while breathing out.

3. When breathing in, you must learn to keep the upper part of the chest still, so that the breathing is performed mainly by the abdominal muscles and diaphragm. When breathing out, the abdominal wall should contract and sink in toward the spine; by allowing the abdominal wall to relax, or sag out, the next breath is drawn into the lungs automatically. All exercises should finish by breathing out with the abdomen contracted.

4. Breathe out sufficiently to hear the wheezing noises in the bases of the lungs. This may cause coughing and increase wheezing, but it should be persevered with gently. Rest for a minute or two before each exercise.

5. To begin with, the exercise should be done very gently, with plenty of rest. When there is "tightness in the chest," do it in the reclining position, that is, lie back on the pillows with your knees bent comfortably.

6. It is a good thing to time with a watch how long you can keep up this blowing out, but on no account must you take a deep breath first. To begin with, a few seconds is all you can do, but, later on, you may be able to sustain the whistle for 40 to 60 seconds.

House Dust Precautions

House dust is not ordinary dirt. It is a substance which forms on the inside of mattresses, pillows, upholstered furniture and other stuffed articles that cannot be washed.

The prevention and control of allergy demands strict attention to the following:

1. The bedroom should contain only one bed and no upholstered furniture.

2. Mattresses and pillows must be encased in allergen-proof covers.

3. No mattress pad may be used. Washable blankets only are to be used for covers.

4. All upholstered furniture in the house must be vacuum-cleaned daily.

5. Keep the bedroom door closed off from the rest of the house.

6. When you get allergen-proof covers, and not before, houseclean the bedroom, take the mattress and pillow outside and do not bring them back into the clean room until they are covered.

7. It is desirable to render the patient's room dust-free. It should be entered seldom by others. All cleaning should be done when the patient is not in the room.

8. Remove all hangings, carpets and extra furnishings from the sleeping room, as these catch dust. There should be no stuffed furniture in the room. Clean the walls and ceilings. Scrub the woodwork, floors and closets. Wax the floors. Scrub the bedsprings.

9. Cover the mattress, pillows and box springs with dustproof covers. Use washable blankets and washable bedspreads.

10. A scrubbed chair may be used. Use rag rugs and plain, light curtains. Wash them weekly.

11. When possible, the ventilation should be obtained from a hallway or another room. If there is sensitivity to wool, ordinary blankets may be put into sheets before being brought into the room. These sheets should be changed only outside the room.

12. Do not store much outer clothing, such as shoes

and overcoats, or other household objects, in the clothes closets.

13. If furnace heat outlets exist, a dust filter must be obtained, installed and changed frequently.

Remember that the carrying out of these precautions is your own responsibility. The doctor's treatment and medicines will be effective only if you cooperate.

Further Important Directions for the Avoidance of House Dust*

House dust is a special substance to which many people become allergic, and is known to be due to the deterioration of various objects, materials and fabrics. Light greyish, usually fuzzy, house dust is to be distinguished from heavier street dust, and is not the same thing. It may be present in abundance in an apparently clean house. Allergy to house dust may cause symptoms at any time of the year and is known to be the main cause of asthma in the winter. The concentration of house dust in the winter is greater because of heavy clothes, rugs, drapes, blankets, closed windows and so forth. A flare-up of symptoms often occurs during the changeable weather of fall and spring.

Treatment or "hyposensitization" (immunization) with an effective extract is extremely important, and will usually give a considerable amount of help. However, it is also necessary for the patient to avoid overexposure, as symptoms may appear at times when he is well under treatment. The treatment gets off to a better start when the person avoids getting too much house dust into his system. THEREFORE, BOTH TREATMENT AND AVOIDANCE ARE TWO IMPORTANT REQUIREMENTS THAT HAVE TO BE

---

* Henry D. Ogden, M.D., New Orleans, Louisiana.

TAKEN CARE OF IN ORDER TO OBTAIN THE
BEST RESULTS. The following suggestions are helpful, and are not as difficult as they seem at first glance.

A PERSON ALLERGIC TO HOUSE DUST OB-
VIOUSLY SHOULD AVOID DUSTY OBJECTS
AND ROOMS, SUCH AS ATTICS, CELLARS AND
STOREROOMS, AND SHOULD AVOID RUM-
MAGING IN BOXES, DRAWERS AND SO FORTH.
It is particularly necessary to cut down the amount of
dust in the bedroom, because here most people spend
eight to 10 hours of the 24. It should be thoroughly
cleaned at least every week by another person, and a
light cleaning should be given every day. To a lesser
degree, the same precautions should be followed for the
rest of the house. A bedroom in the middle of a long,
one-story house is really only one section of a longer
room. In this type of home, the whole dwelling must
receive particular attention. If possible, the dust-allergic
person should have a room which is well ventilated and
connected by a door with the rest of the house.

The walls, floor and ceiling of the bedroom must be
carefully cleaned, and particular attention must be paid
to the windows, venetian blinds, molding, backs and
tops of pictures, drawers in dressers, tops of doors, backs
and undersides of furniture and so forth. It is really
better to remove each object from the room and return
it only after it has been thoroughly cleaned. The bedsprings must be washed. Hard surfaces, furniture, cop-
ings, springs, venetian blinds and so forth should be
waxed or gone over with an oiled cloth. Linoleum rugs
or floors may be waxed, or at least kept scrupulously
clean. Throw rugs may be used if they are washed
frequently.

There should be no storage in the room of the patient. Such things as sweaters, shoes, books, pictures,

magazines and knickknacks must be kept in another part of the house. The room should contain only those objects which are needed and which are, more or less, in frequent use. If there is a closet, it must be kept absolutely clean and the door must be kept shut. All cracks or holes in the walls, floor or ceiling should be sealed.

AS DUST WILL FORM IN MATTRESSES AND PILLOWS, IT IS NECESSARY FOR THE PATIENT TO SECURE SPECIAL DUSTPROOF COVERS FOR ALL MATRESSES, PILLOWS AND BOX SPRINGS IN THE ROOM. Your allergist can tell you where such covers may be obtained. It is better to put on these covers outside the bedroom. Covers made of ordinary cloth material are not satisfactory, and plastic covers with zippers are not particularly recommended.

The bed should not have a mattress pad unless it is washed frequently, and comforters should not be used. Chenille spreads or any fuzzy material may form or collect dust. It is good to use a sheet on both sides of the blankets, which should be washed at frequent intervals. Soft, upholstered furniture must be removed or covered and sealed with a dustproof material. Plastic or leather furniture, which may be easily cleaned, is definitely preferable. It is a good idea to avoid sitting on uncovered, overstuffed furniture or on uncovered pillows. Foam rubber mattresses, pillows or furniture are satisfactory; these may also be covered if desired. If there is more than one bed in the patient's bedroom, the others should also be dustproofed. Incidentally, if foam rubber mattresses are used, the box springs must be properly covered.

Curtains, rugs and blankets must be washable, and must be washed at frequent intervals. Also, all clothing used must be either washed or dry-cleaned frequently. Such cleaning is especially necessary for clothes that have been stored for a time, even though the clothes have been wrapped up or protected. This is particularly true in the fall of the year. Unused clothing is best kept in another part of the house. It is, therefore, better to dress and undress in another room.

The use of a vacuum cleaner is helpful for general housecleaning. It is especially helpful to clean wallpaper. The patient must always be out of the house when any cleaning is going on, and the bedroom may be aired for several hours after cleaning. Housewives who are allergic to house dust must arrange for someone else to do the actual housecleaning. If it is necessary to do cleaning, a mask should be worn. If the patient is a child, stuffed or "dust-catching" toys should not be used. Pets should not be allowed in the house.

A temporary flare-up of symptoms may occur at times after visiting certain dusty places, such as some theaters, hotels, offices and warehouses. Temperature or weather changes often affect an allergic person, and an otherwise comfortable patient may occasionally have trouble during cooler or wet weather or during weather changes. Therefore, marked changes in temperature should be guarded against. The sleeping room should be well aired, but must be kept warm in cool weather. The patient should, if possible, not have his bed next to the window if it is used for ventilation.

A floor furnace is good, but, if this is not practical, an ordinary gas stove or electric heater may be used. The temperature should not be allowed to go below 72 degrees Fahrenheit. Some hot air systems are bad. A filtered warm air heating system is good. Such a system may be arranged to furnish heat in the winter and air in the summer. If there is an unfiltered central heating unit, outlets should be covered with coarse muslin.

True respiratory infections or "colds" may also cause

a flare-up of symptoms. On the other hand, many so-called "colds" are pure and simple flare-ups of the allergic condition itself. This is one reason why "colds" are so often helped by tablets for allergy (antihistamines). Occasionally, low-grade fever may accompany such a flare-up. In a true infection, the patient may be quite toxic, have considerable fever and so forth, or *both* allergy and infection may be active at the same time in the same individual.

Mold and Mildew

What is mildew? Molds grow on anything that causes mildew from which they get enough food—cellulose products like cotton, linen, wood and paper, and protein substances like silk and wool.

Where does mildew come from? The molds are always present in the air, but need moisture and certain temperatures in order to grow. Molds commonly develop in muggy summer weather, especially if the house has been closed. They flourish wherever it is damp, warm, poorly aired and poorly lighted—in closets, on shower doors, in damp clothes rolled up for ironing. Also, molds are likely to grow in a newly-built house because of moisture in the building materials.

Is mildew harmful? Yes, it will discolor fabrics and leather, leave a musty odor, decay wood and sometimes so severely eat into cloth that it rots and falls to pieces. It may cause severe allergy.

How can you prevent mildew? Keep things clean. Dust that settles on articles can supply sufficient food for mildew to start. Keep things aired and dry. In rainy weather, keep things as dry as possible. Close doors and windows if it is warm and damp outside. Warm, moist air coming in condenses on colder surfaces of the house, and creates a cool, dry atmosphere inside. As the cool air is warmed inside, the musty air will absorb the moisture. Poorly ventilated closets become damp and musty during continued wet weather, and clothing hung in them is likely to mildew. To dry the air, burn a small electric light continuously in the closet. The heat is enough to stop mildew if the space is not too large. Leave closet doors and dresser drawers open occasionally to keep moisture from gathering and to stir up the enclosed air. Take special care to ventilate linen closets. Run an electric fan in places that cannot be exposed to air. Never let damp or wet clothing lie around. Dry soiled clothes before throwing them into the hamper, stretch out shower curtains to dry. Clean or wash clothing items before storing. Do not leave sizing or laundry starch in fabrics to be stored, because molds feed on these finishes. From time to time, sun and air garments stored in closets. Put away woolen clothing in garment bags.

To protect leather against mildew, sponge with a one per cent solution of paranitrophenol (available at drugstores) in alcohol. To be sure it does not change the color of the leather, test a small area where it will not show. Paranitrophenol protects against mildew for two or three months. Thymol is another chemical that can be used in the same way (one per cent solution in alcohol). Protect leather shoes with a good wax dressing. And don't forget the soles.

For painted surfaces, you can make a mildew-resistant paint by replacing 20 per cent or more of the regular pigment with zinc oxide, for a mildew-resistant finish for outdoor wood surfaces, and spar varnish to exterior oil paint, but only with dark colors.

To keep books in closed bookcases from mildewing, dust them at times with paraformaldehyde. Use this chemical sparingly, for it may be irritating. Another way is to burn a small electric light continuously in the bookcase. To remove mildew from textiles, remove textiles as soon as mildew is discovered, before the growth has a chance to weaken or rot material. Brush off the growth outdoors to prevent scattering the spores in the house.

To remove mildew from fresh stains, wash at once with soap and water, rinse and dry in the sun. If stains remain, moisten with lemon juice and salt, and put in the sun to bleach. To remove mildew from old stains, dip them in Javelle water or other chlorine bleach for no longer than one minute. Then dip into a weak vinegar solution (two tablespoons to each cup of water) to stop action of chlorine. Finally, rinse well. Never use a chlorine bleach on silk or wool. On leather, wipe with a cloth wrung out of diluted alcohol (one cup of denatured alcohol to one cup of water). Dry in a current of air. To remove mildew from floors and woodwork, wipe with a cloth dipped in water to which at little kerosene has been added. Remove mildew stains from painted surfaces with commercial paint remover.

Feather and Kapok Avoidance*

Feathers and kapok are equally common irritants. A person sensitive to either must avoid every possible contact with both.

Canaries, pigeons, parrots or fowl may be the source of feather irritation. It is best to dispose of them. However, the greatest source of feather and kapok contact is bedding—pillows, mattresses, box springs, comforters, quilts, cushions, upholstered furniture and so forth.

Elimination of feathers and kapok can be accom-

---

* Granted for use by Allergy-Free Products for the Home.

plished in two ways: by ridding your home of the articles in which they are present, or by rendering those articles dustproof. (Some kinds of kapok break into minute particles of dust and should be replaced.)

Ordinary feather and kapok pillows may be dustproofed by covering them with individually sized Protecto-Dust casings. These casings remain dustproof and comfortable after wear and washings. Since no zippers are airtight, there are deep, wide flaps extending well beyond the ends of the lifetime zippers to prevent dust seepage. Feather and down cushions and mattresses should be replaced with smooth-surface latex foam plus Protecto-Dust casings.

The reason a feather or down cushion needs to be replaced is because it bears the whole weight of the body —the compression is too great. A feather pillow holds only the weight of the head and can be encased.

Comforters and quilts should be discarded in favor of no-fuzz 100 per cent cotton blankets and no-fuzz 100 per cent wool blankets that have been washed and treated. If this is not possible, get a nylon-coated or 200 count (not less) percale blanket cover. Coated nylon tends to slip—it needs to be tucked in or used with blanket clips. A washable electric sheet (not blanket) may be used.

Now a word of caution. The plastic bedding covers that are sold in stores are not sufficiently dustproof. Latex foam, dacron and acrilan pillows should have Protecto-Dust casings.

By following these simple instructions, the home will not only be free of feather and kapok sources, but all future cleanings will be much easier and faster.

However, it is necessary to be mindful of possible contacts while visiting, shopping or in business.

Animal Hairs and Danders

Many vareties of animal hair, dander or fur are responsible for inhalant allergy. Occasionally, the etiologic relationship is hard to trace. The following animal danders are most commonly found in the home: cat, dog, horse, cow, goat, rabbit, camel and muskrat.

Horse Dander: Not many allergic people react to horse dander. Horse dander, however, is one of the most common manifestations of allergy to animal hairs. Horse dander sensitive patients should not be treated with sera of equine origin, unless they are carefully desensitized. Horsehair is contained in mattresses, pillows, upholstery, felts and fabric blankets, and is used especially in the padding of coats, the lining of shoes, gloves, brushes, sacks, bags, rope, wigs and pony hair coats. It is often used to stuff and cover furniture of the mid-Victorian period. Dander and airborne emanations arise from hair mattresses and cloth as they age in wear. The dust that accumulates in furniture stuffed with horsehair will often produce severe reactions. Workers in shops which use uncleaned hair, hostlers, horsemen, horse fanciers and farmers are especially apt to develop severe allergy. Emanations of mules, donkeys and, to a less extent, of other mammalian animals are also apt to affect horse dander sensitive patients. The effect of manure on lawns or streets, especially in countries where horses or mules are still used, is to be recognized. Proximity to barns, fields or tracks where there are horses affects sensitive patients. People who are violently sensitive to horse dander should not visit buildings where horses are used and where they are shown.

Cats and Dogs: These animals are especially apt to produce sensitizations. It is not sufficient for a cat or dog asthmatic or allergic person to avoid contact with these animals. The animals should be kept out of the house at all times. Accumulated evidence indicates that de-sensitization to one species will not produce satisfactory protection to all. Allergy to these animals often requires the most careful elimination of their emanations from rooms, furnitures, carpets and over the basements and yards of the patient's home. Sometimes, families will object to removing their pet dogs or cats. A trial period of six to eight weeks away from the dogs or cats usually convinces most patients that it is better to be asthma- or rhinitis-free than to retain the pet and continue to suffer. The use of the pelts of these animals in cheap furs must be remembered. One patient was sensitive to cat hair and had a violent conjunctival reaction when one hair from a cheap fur, worn by a woman in front of her in a theatre, lodged in her eye. Cat hair is put into some bedding and furniture, according to Thoma. Its skin may be used to line coats, gloves, caps or shoes, or may be used in robes. The close relation of fox, coyote and wolf to dog and cat indicates the consideration of allergy from rugs, robes and coats from such animals in dog- and cat-sensitive patients. Dog hair is used at times with wool in Chinese rugs. The saliva, or the scratch or the hair contact of these animals may produce urticaria or dermatitis in patients sensitive to the emanations.

Cattle Hair: Tests with cattle or cow hair should be routine. It, and other animal hair, enters the composition of pads under carpets, especially of Ozite, and it is incorporated in cheap blankets, robes, carpets, upholstery, felt, brushes, certain Chinese rugs and cheap building felt; it is also mixed with horsehair in blankets and mattresses. Calf skin is used in coats and as covering for furniture. The extensive use of leather, and allergies arising among workers of this product, is interesting. Farmers, cattlemen, butchers and so forth are especially apt to develop cattle hair allergies.

Rabbit Hair: Rabbit hair is the origin of several allergic reactions in certain patients. Reactions from rabbit hair used as fur are not uncommon. Breeders and men handling the animals may be sensitized. Rabbit hair is often found in mattresses, quilts, pillows, cushions, linings of gloves and shoes, cuffs, collars, cheap furs and toys. It is the main ingredient in felt used in hats. The great use of Angora rabbit fur in the fur industry is noteworthy. As a yarn, it is used often with silk to make infants' wear, underwear, hosiery, trimmings and other wearing apparel.

Camel Hair: Camel hair is a source of definite allergy in keepers of such animals. It produces allergy in the public occasionally because of its use in coats, sweaters, shawls, rugs, felt, blankets, brushes, certain fabrics, linings and boltings. It is used in Oriental rugs and to make Jaeger cloth and under garments.

Hog Hair: Hog hair allergy may develop in men handling the animals or their hides. The hair is sometimes used in furniture, cushions and, especially, in mattresses and brushes.

Guinea Pig: Guinea pig emanation frequently sensitizes animal workers. A case of this was first reported in 1868. One patient was known later to be so sensitive that an exposure of a few minutes produced asthma, which gradually disappeared in five days.

Goat Hair Allergy: Goat hair is being used more extensively, and becomes a definite cause of allergy. Mohair from Angora goats is utilized in plushes, coat linings, summer suits, rugs, curtains, cloth, horse blankets, muffs, brushes, robes, curtain braids and trimmings, wigs, doll hair and, especially, in upholstery of furniture and automobiles. Italians also use it in bedding. The wool of Cashmere goats is made into shawls and alpaca, and that of Peruvian goats into alpaca and yarns used in certain fabrics. Skins with the hair are used for coats, muffs, capes and automobile robes. The fine wool is woven into Oriental rugs. Goat herders and those who merchandise the crude hair and make it into the commercial articles indicated above are apt to be sensitized.

Sheep Wool Allergy: Sheep wool is used more extensively in carpets, clothes and furnishings than is any other animal hair. It frequently is responsible for allergy, but, fortunately, rarely produces severe manifestations that can compare to those arising from horse dander. Wool clothing, however, frequently produces skin allergy, and is responsible for some generalized pruritus. When well brushed and made of fine fibers, wool is not especially productive of bronchial allergy, as reported by Korn and many others. Wool in clothing, however, should not be brushed in the patient's room. Patients moderately sensitive to wool usually can tolerate well-washed, nonfuzzy woolen blankets, especially as desensitization progresses. Some very sensitive patients, however, cannot inhale any wool allergen without exaggeration of symptoms. This demands elimination of all wool from the environment until desensitization is effective.

In addition, sheep wool is used as a filling for quilts and mattresses and in paddings, clothes, tapestry, furniture and robes. Sheepskin coats and gloves and other articles made from the hides, many of which have the wool on their inner surfaces, cause some disturbances. The methods of environmental control and therapy are the same as already described. The following commercial materials contain wool: albatross, astrakhan, chinchilla, broadcloth, carpets, cheviot, cravenette, doeskin, felt, flannel, wool gabardine, homespun jersey, mackinaw, melton, poplin, rugs, serge, suede cloth, tapestry, mohair (imitation), tweed, velour, whipcord, worsted, padding for robes and mattresses, quilts and wool for medical purposes. Cloaks of varying types, felts and many other materials are made from wool and used in hundreds of ways in industry. The use of wool grease as lanolin in soap, ointments and creams is not to be forgotten.

Pyrethrum

Pyrethrum is contained in most insecticides, either in the form of powders or sprays. Patients, sensitized to this allergen, often have asthma or nasal symptoms in public places, such as theaters or hotels, because of the use of pyrethrum in insecticides and moth exterminators in the carpets, furniture and curtains.

Pyrethrum is the most common constituent of insect powders and sprays. It is derived from the dried, powdered flower of the pyrethrum plant. Botanically, pyrethrum is a member of the chrysanthemum family.

Individuals who react to pyrethrum extract will usually react to chrysanthemum extract.

Pyrethrum is a common sensitizer, and it is often responsible for symptoms in those who are sensitive to it. Pyrethrum is found in the following nationally advertised insecticides: Flit, Black Flag, Gulf Spray and many types of aerosol bombs.

It is often found in combination with DDT. Pyrethrum, on occasions, is also incorporated in medicines, as ointments and solutions, and is used to treat parastic infections of the human skin. Occasionally, it has also been used in medicines administered internally for the treatment of intestinal parasites.

It is mostly used to mothproof new and old carpets, draperies and upholsteries, and to prevent the growth of various other insects in these materials. It is also used in theatres, churches and other public places for the elimination of insects.

One can usually avoid pyrethrum easily at home. It is more difficult to avoid it away from home. Pyrethrum allergy usually occurs during those months when insects are most prevalent. It will be necessary for you to take hyposensitization treatment with an extract prepared from pyrethrum, if you are sensitive to pyrethrum and work in a public building where pyrethrum-containing insecticides are constantly being used.

As a substitute for pyrethrum for killing insects, you may use the following preparations:

Kilit (Lancaster Allergy Supply Company, Lancaster, Pennsylvania)

Cederene (Allergy Free Products, 226 Livingston Street, Brooklyn, New York)

If you use DDT, be sure that the preparation you buy is not mixed with pyrethrum.

Orris Root

Orris root consists of the pulverized root of several varieties of iris grown in southern Europe. The oil and fine starch granules hold the perfume. Because of this and its faint violet odor, it is often used in cosmetic powders and toilet articles.

Cosmetics

Face powders	Perfumes
Shaving cream	Lipstick
Facial creams	Scented soaps
Tooth powder	Teething rings
Sunburn lotion	Bath salts
Sachets	Toothpaste
Shampoos	Hair tonic
Rouges	

Tincture of orris is used in cosmetics; hence, some products contain orris when they do not have any powdered orris root in them.

Contacts

The most common is through the use of the products listed above. Other contacts are at parties, churches and theaters. If others in the household use orris, you cannot avoid it.

Treatment

Discard your old powder puff. Eliminate from your home every product containing orris root. Do not allow the barber to use any powder on you. Desensitization to orris is necessary, and should be continued at least a year or longer.

Substitution

Cosmetics are never truly "nonallergic," but these are free of orris root* and may be used:

Elizabeth Arden	Armand's Symphony
Marcelle	Botay
Mary-Dunhill	Max Factor's Pancake
Ar-Ex	Almay
Allercreme	

---

* This report does not necessarily mean other products may not be free of orris root, but assurance should be obtained before using.

It is best to use the nonscented forms of the brand you select!

Directions for the Avoidance of Orris Root

If you are sensitive to orris root, you should use no scented soaps, scented tooth powders or mouth washes, bath salts, perfumes, cleansing creams or cosmetics concerning which you are uncertain as to orris root content. Of course everything that is perfumed does not necessarily contain orris root. But one who is allergic to orris root must know positively that any particular substance does not. Most perfumes and cosmetics are made with secret formulas, and the manufacturers of cosmetics are sometimes unwilling to list the ingredients. Fortunately, however, several manufacturers of cosmetics have been willing to cooperate with allergists in the manufacture of high-grade cosmetics which are free from orris root.

Unscented body talcs, such as Squibb or Colgate Unscented, usually do not contain orris root.

Orris root is sometimes used in shampoos in beauty parlors.

One may be exposed to orris root, even through one does not wear cosmetics. A child may be exposed to those worn by his mother or his nurse. Such persons also should wear cosmetics which do not contain orris root. A man using talc after shaving may have symptoms from orris root, or after the reasonably close exposure that exists at a dance or in a movie or church social. Occasionally, especially if there are several women in a family, orris root becomes pretty well distributed through the dust of a house. Bridge parties and the like may result in contact with this substance, even though the patient does not expose himself intentionally.

Therefore, for best results, desensitization, as well as avoidance, is sometimes required.

You should bear in mind that cosmetics which do not contain orris root contain other substances, such as rice powder or oatmeal powder, to which you might be sensitive. If, therefore, your symptoms continue in spite of treatment, it will be necessary to test you with the orris root-free cosmetics which you will be using.

Orris root powder or oil is commonly found in face powders, sachets, perfumes, bath salts, facial cream, scented soaps, toothpaste and powders and hair tonics. Control requires the thorough eradication of orris-containing products from the patient's environment. Thus, the closets, medicine cabinets, bureau and wardrobe drawers, suitcases and trunks which have contained such materials or clothes, or fabrics which might hold even slight traces of orris root products, should be thoroughly cleaned or renovated. It must be emphasized that the patient's clothes, furs, collars, pillows, mattresses and bedding may also hold enough orris allergen to produce symptoms in a very sensitive individual.

Flaxseed*

The Latin word "linum," from which our word "linen" is derived, means "flax." Flaxseed is the seed of the flax plant. Skin reactions to flaxseed are fairly common, and this substance should be avoided by individuals who have positive skin tests and by those who know that they have trouble from this substance. Flaxseed may be the cause of a reaction when taken as a food (ingestant or inhaled as a dust (inhalant) or by direct

---

* Granted for use by Hollister-Stier Laboratories (Flaxseed, karaya gum, orris root and cottonseed avoidance) .

contact with the skin (contactant). A person sensitive
to flaxseed should avoid it in every form.

Ingestants

Cereals: Roman meal and Uncle Sam's Breakfast Food

Flaxseed tea

Flaxolyn—a laxative

Milk of cows fed flaxseed (causes reactions in very sensitive persons)

Flaxseed extracts used occasionally in cough remedies

Inhalants and Contactants

Flaxseed meal as a food for cattle and poultry

Flaxseed used in poultry tonics

Wavesets, shampoos and hair tonics which contain flaxseed (Kremel)

Bird lime

Flaxseed poultices

Linseed oil

Linoleum (Latin meaning flax oil)—dust from linoleum may cause symtoms

Carron oil

Furniture polish

Paints and varnishes

Printers' and lithographic ink

Soft Soap

Depilatories (some)'

Cloth Materials

(rarely cause trouble, except when very coarse or in cases of extreme sensitivity)

Art linen

Damask

Bird's eye (linen)

Table linen

Handkerchief linen

Huckaback

Sewing thread

Sheeting

Dress linen

Cambric

Toweling

Collars and cuffs

Oilcloth

Miscellaneous

Insulating material—Flaxlinum used in refrigerators Bi-flax, a base used for insulating plaster

Rugs (Klear flax)

Straw mats

Paper—high-grade wax paper as stuffing material for furniture upholstery, chair seats, cushions and so forth

Fiberboard

Flaxseed Allergy

Flaxseed may produce dermatitis, cutaneous edema
and gastrointestinal symptoms, in addition to asthma.

Flaxseed allergen may be found in all food meals for stock and in chicken food; shampoos and, especially, wavesets; paints which contain linseed oil; varnishes; polishes; soap; carron oil; linoleum and oilcloth. The rare patient may be so sensitive as to make it essential to eliminate fabrics containing flax, such as art linen, bird's eye linen, cambric, damask, linen huckaback, sheeting, toweling, collars and cuffs. This flaxseed alergen may also be found in poultices, flaxseed tea, wadding, Roman meal and linen cloth. Linseed oil, which is contained in furniture polish and paints, is. made from flaxseed. This may be an explanation of the violent bronchial reactions some patients have to the smell of such material.

Patients have been noted to have asthma from hair spray. The ingestion of Roman meal has been known to cause asthma. When such sensitivity exists, the removel of all flaxseed from medicine closets should be insisted upon.

Silk Allergy

Silk allergy is not uncommon. Dust from silk curtains, garments, upholstery and covers is present in many homes and public places, and incorporates itself in house dust.

Allergy to silk usually occurs from contact with silk, as most often seen in the skin either as an urticaria or atopic dermatitis, and less often as a contact dermatitis. At times, silk is responsible for inhalant symptoms, and may cause asthma and allergic coryza.

Investigations by other workers in the field of allergy have revealed that the major portion of contact dermatitis attributed to silk is usually due to some other constituent of the cloth, such as the plastic coating used to enhance the sheen, or to the dye in the cloth.

Vaughan found that silk caused atopic dermatitis more frequently than contact dermatitis, presumably due to the inhalation of the excitant.

Silk-sensitive patients suffering from atopic dermatitis would have exacerbations of their dermatitis if they wore silk. Persons allergic to silk usually react severely to extremely high dilutions. Silk is found in the following: broadcloth, silk brocade, Canton crepe, silk casement cloths, chiffon, China silk, crepe de Chine, duchess satin, foulard, faille, georgette, taffeta, jersey, plush, pongee, rugs, silk poplin, radium silk, ribbons, wash satin, tub silk, tulle, thread, upholstery and tapestries, velvets, silk floss for lining, knit goods, hosiery, mufflers, cheap silk neckties, pillows and so forth. Many fabrics with trade names and different yarns and threads also contain varying amounts of silk.

Karaya Gum Allergy

Karaya gum is used as a substitute for tragacanth and acacia gum. It is obtained from several East Indian trees of the genus *Stericula*. Karaya gum is also known under the name gum arabic.

Karaya gum is found in the following:

Drugs

Bassoran (Merrell)	Imbicol (Upjohn)

Denture Adhesive Powders

Dr. Werner's Powder	Stix
Dent-a-Firm	Nyko Adherent Powder
Denture Powder	

Toothpastes

Lactona	Listerine

Hair-fixing Solutions

Karaba	Karabim (G. A. Brown & Company)
Kara Jel	Mucara (Upjohn)

Foods

Diabetic foods, including soybean and almond wafers

Certain brands of gelatin and Junket

Commercially prepared ices, ice creams, flavors, emulsions and some salad dressings

Fillers for lemon, custard and other factory-made pies

Some brands of ice cream and ice cream liquid mix

Gum drops and similar candies

Prepared ice cream powders

Commercial

Many emulsified mineral oils and laxatives

Many hand lotions (Saraka)

Karaya gum is also used as an offset material in printing inks, wall-fixing solutions and adhesives

Gum arabic has also been used for intravenous infusion

Knox gelatin has no gum in it

Glue Allergy

Allergy to glue, when it occurs, is very severe. Desensitization should begin with very dilute extracts.

Feinberg lists the following uses of glue: by cabinet workers and carpenters, on envelope flaps, in the making of pads and books, on sandpaper and matches, labels, gummed paper, court plasters, in sizing cloth and paper, in the preparation of gelatin, jellies and isinglass and in combs and buttons. It is also used in mucilages and pastes. Dust from glue used in furniture and books is often encountered in homes and, especially, in libraries. Reactions have been reported in glue-sensitive patients wearing shoes with innersoles glued therein. Children may be affected from the use of glue in stamp-collecting or kite or airplane-making.

Cottonseed*

Cottonseed may be contacted in any of these forms:

Linters: Linters is the name given to the short fibers

---

* Granted for use by Hollister-Stier Laboratories.

that cling to the cottonseeds after the long fibers have been removed. These linters contain fragments of the seeds. They are used in spinning or in making cotton wadding or batting. Wadding or batting is used to make pads and cushions, comforters, some mattresses and upholstery; these things made of batting or wadding should not be used by cottonseed-allergic people. Methods for avoiding contacts with mattresses and upholstery are given in the house dust instructions.

Varnishes, particularly those used for coating metals, artificial leather and waterproofing, are often made from linters; hence, wet varnishes should be avoided.

Cottonseed Meal Products: Cottonseed cake and meal are used as fertilizer, feed for cattle, poultry, horses, hogs and sheep. The flour is used for human food. It is used sometimes to make gin. It is also used to make xylose or wood sugar. Xylose has a sweet taste and may be used in soft drinks, but, to our knowledge, it is not used in the common soft drinks. Be sure to watch for and avoid all these contacts!

*Cottonseed Oil***:* The finest cottonseed oil is used for food. Most salad oils contain this oil, as do most oleomargarines. Mayonnaises and salad dressings are almost always made with cottonseed oil. Lard compounds and lard substitutes are made with cottonseed oil. You should avoid all these products.

Sardines may be packed in cottonseed oil. Most commercial frying and baking of cakes, breads, fish, popcorn, potato chips and doughnuts is also done with cottonseed oil. This oil is used almost universally in restaurants. Thus, you must eat at home or at places that do

*** The incidence of allergenic substance in cottonseed oil and its products is debatable. This listing is given to show the many uses it has and the many things to be considered when it is recommended that all contact with cottonseed be avoided.

not use cottonseed. Pure lard and corn oil may be used in your cooking.

Candies, particularly chocolate, often contain cottonseed oil. Find out from your confectioner which candies are free of this oil. Olive oil is often adulterated with cottonseed oil. It is used as a base for liniments and salves. Camphorated oil and miners' and alter lamps may contain cottonseed oil.

It is also used in the manufacture of paper, salt, machine tools and paint. You should avoid industrial shops where fumes of cottonseed may be inhaled.

Cottonseed is used in some cosmetics. Avoid using such brands.

Cottonseed oil is used to polish fruit at fruit stands. Check for this!

Both cottonseed and flaxseed are excreted in the milk of animals. Because these seeds are often fed to cattle, you will have to omit milk if you cannot get it from animals not fed cottonseed or flaxseed

Cottonseed Oil Products*

SHORTENINGS	OLEOMARGARINES	SALAD OILS
Advance	Meadowlake	Wesson Oil
Bakerite	Cotton Blossom	Winco
Mrs. Tucker's	Allsweet	Mrs. Tucker's
Scoco	Nucoa	Contadina
Jasimine	Dixie	Jewel Oil
Creamtex	Good Luck	Margherita
Humko		Crustene
Jewel		Esskay
Snowdrift		Armour's Star
Crisco		Magnolia
Flako		
Armour's Vegetole		

* This is a partial list of shortenings, oleomargarines and salad oils.

Mayonnaise

These and many others are made with cottonseed oil:
Good Luck, Hellman's, Best Foods and Durkee's.

Cottonseed Allergy

INGESTANTS:

Salad oils
Lard substitutes
Butter substitutes
Sardines (packing oil)
Olives (setting solution)
Bakery goods
Confectionery coating to
 hold chocolate firm
Wesson oil, a pure grade cot-
 tonseed oil
Crisco, hardened cottonseed
 oil or Spry
Cottolene, beef suet and cot-
 tonseed oil
Oleomargarines (most)

CONTACTANTS:

Cosmetics
Olive oil substitute (used in
 the compounding of emul-
 sions)

Liniment base
Salves
Camphorated oil

INHALANTS:

Mattresses
Pillows
Cotton blankets
Stuffing in furniture
Greens and fairways in mini-
 ature golf courses
Cattle food

MATERIALS IN WAVESET
LOTIONS:

Flaxseed
India gum
Acacia
Quince seed

Soybean*

Soybeans have been grown in Asia for centuries, especially in China. To the Orientals, they have been
bread, meat and oil. Since 1804, American farmers have
grown soybeans and fed them to livestock or plowed
them under for fertilizer. In the last few years, the
chemists have found many uses for this lowly bean, and
soybeans are proving to be a treasure and a bonanza.

---

* Granted for use by Hollister-Stier Laboratories.

Foods

1. *Bakery Goods.* Soybean flour containing only 1 per cent oil is now used by many bakers in their dough mixtures for breads, rolls, cakes and pastries. This keeps them moist and salable several days longer. The roasted nuts are used in place of peanuts. K-biscuits and several crisp crackers have soybean flour in them.

2. *Sauces:* Oriental Show You Sauce, Lea & Perrins Sauce, La Choy Sauce, Heinz Worcestershire Sauce.

3. *Cereals:* Sunlets (American Dietaids Company, Yonkers, New York). Cellu Soy Flakes (Chicago Dietetic Supply House, Chicago, Illinois)

4. *Salad Dressing:* E-P-K French Dressing (Price Flavoring & Extract Company, Chicago, Illinois)

Many of the salad dressings and mayonnaises contain soy oil but only state on the label that they contain vegetable oil. Present conditions have necessitated the use of soy oil in many brands of oil previously free of soybean.

5. *Meats:* Pork link sausage and lunch meats may contain soybeans.

6. *Candies:* Soy flour is used in hard candies, nut candies and caramels. Lecithin is invariably derived from soybean, and is used in candies to prevent drying out and to emulsify the fats.

7. *Milk Substitutes:* Sobee (Mead Johnson & Company), Mull-Soy (Borden Company). Some bakeries use soy milk instead of cow's milk.

8. Ice Cream

9. Joy Anna (A. Dietaids Company)

10. Soups

11. Vegetables (Fresh soy sprouts are served as a vegetable, especially in Chinese dishes.)

12. Nuts (Soys are roasted, salted and used instead of peanuts.)
13. Soybean noodles, macaroni and spaghetti
14. Reezon seasoning (A. Dietaids Company)
15. Crisco, Spry and other shortenings
16. Oleomargarine and butter substitutes
17. Cheese Tufu, Natto and Miso, as well as some others

Contacts

Varnish	Paper sizing	Custards
Candles	Paper finishes	Textile dressing
Linoleum	Automobile parts	Lubricating oil
Nitroglycerine	Glycerine	Printing ink
Soap	Illuminating oil	Massage creams
Fodder	Enamels	Grease
Coffee subsitutes	Cloth	Gro-Pup dog food
Paints	Adhesives	French's fish food
Celluloid	Blankets	

New Contacts

Many new contacts are to be expected. If you remember that soybeans are used as flour, oil, milk and nuts, it will be possible to anticipate most new contacts.

25 *Diets, Aids and Recipes**

THE EXISTENCE of peculiar, abnormal reactions, or idio-syncrasies, to foods has been recognized since ancient times. Only within comparatively recent years, however, have reactions been proved to be due to hypersensitive-ness, or allergy, to these foods. Such hypersensitiveness has been found capable of provoking practically any type of clinical manifestation of allergy, except that due to pollen. The exact incidence of food allergy is difficult to determine, because it is not always easy to prove a distinct causal relationship.

As in other allergic conditions, hereditary predisposi-tion may play an important role and be responsible for the production of a high degree of sensitivity, which may manifest itself by severe reactions upon contact with the allergen. Hereditary transmission of sensitivity to specific foods may likewise occur. Sensitization to foods also can be acquired; this is true, for example, of urticaria. This type is likely to be less acute and of more temporary character than those with an atopic type of reaction.

Almost any type of food allergen is capable of pro-ducing an allergic reaction. Wheat, milk and eggs are

* Material in this chapter has been taken from the textbook on allergy by Dr. Louis Tuft with his permission.

the most frequent offenders because of their almost universal employment in the diet. Proof of a specific relationship of certain food allergens in the production of symptoms is hampered somewhat by the fact that positive skin reactions are not always accompanied by circulating antibodies; also, proof is hampered by the fact that extracts are prepared in the raw state, whereas the food proteins are subjected, before producing symptoms, to processes of cooking or digestion which may alter or split the protein. Finally, negative skin reaction may occur, even in the presence of definite clinical sensitivity. Group reactions frequently occur with the food allergens.

The clinical manifestations of food allergy already described include allergic coryza, asthma and certain instances of bronchitis, gastrointestinal or abdominal manifestations, urticaria, angioneurotic edema, eczema, dermatitis, migraine and other types of neurologic symptoms and a number of conditions in which the association is considerably less definite and, possibly, open to question. The symptoms of food allergy, therefore, will depend largely upon the type of clinical manifestation produced. The onset of these symptoms may be acute and severe in the highly sensitive and, usually, atopic types, or gradual and less acute in the less sensitive acquired types. Recurrence of attacks is common, as is also the association of more than one clinical manifestation of symptom with the action of a single allergen.

The diagnosis of food allergy is dependent upon history, allergic tests and therapeutic or clinical trial. The history is important when the patient can suspect certain foods as being responsible for attacks, or can supply a history of definite food dislikes. Skin tests are often of invaluable aid in determining the specific exciting factor or factors; they are, however, not infrequently negative, in spite of the presence of definite clinical sensitivity. For this reason, the intracutaneous technique should be used whenever possible. The indirect method of testing by means of passive transfer may be used when the direct method cannot be used satisfactorily.

The method of clinical or therapeutic trial is quite important in food allergy, both because of the necessity of proving the etiologic specificity of foods incriminated by skin tests and, also, because of the necessity of determining the specific factor in patients giving negative skin reactions. For the latter purpose, the use of trial or elimination diets, such as those suggested by Rowe, are very helpful and convenient. Another method of determining food specificity, which may be of value in selected cases, in spite of the tediousness of its technique, is the determination of the leukopenic index. The occurrence of a low white blood cell count after the ingestion of a specific food is evidence of the causative importance of this food.

The treatment of food allergy consists chiefly in the complete elimination from the diet of those foods to which the patient is found specifically sensitive. When the eliminated food is essential to the diet (egg, milk or wheat), attempts at substitution, either by a different food or by altering its specificity, may be tried. If this fails, or when it is desired to restore the food to the diet, methods of desensitization should be attempted. This is done preferably by the oral method, the principle being similar to that of any other type of desensitization. The smallest tolerated dose is given first, and is increased gradually, according to the patient's tolerance. The indications and methods of nonspecific desensitization or of symptomatic treatment are similar to that of any other type, and are dependent to some extent upon the clinical manifestation present.

Finally, in considering the mechanisms by which allergic reactions to foods are produced, it must be emphasized that they are subject to the same principles which govern the production of allergic reactions resulting from any other type of allergen. The influence of heredity, the importance of contact, the role of the serum antibodies and the existence of both inherited and acquired types of sensitization are all well-established facts in relationship to food allergy. Because food allergens enter the tissues through the gastrointestinal tract and, therefore, are subjected to processes of digestion, intestinal absorption and the effect of the liver before entering the general circulation, some discussion has arisen concerning the extent of these influences in the mechanism of the allergic reaction to the food. Extensive experimental investigation has shown that small amounts of unaltered protein can pass through the intestinal wall of normal individuals without causing any disturbance because they are readily disposed of by the liver. However, in previously sensitized individuals, allergic reactions may be provoked by this absorption. Furthermore, food ingested by individuals with normal digestion is so transformed that it does not contain any protein molecules which are not broken down into amino acid. In individuals with food allergy, this transformation is incomplete; insufficently modified proteins pass through the liver, enter the blood stream and provoke allergic reactions in the sensitized patient. One would suspect that, on the basis of such a conception of the pathogenesis, food allergy should be more common. However, from experiments in animals, it would appear that continued ingestion of the foods tends to

*Wheat**

establish an immunity, and that sensitization occurs only when the allergic reaction overcomes the antagonistic process of immunity.

Wheat is found in the following foods:

1. *Beverages:* Cocomalt, beer,** gin (any drink containing grain neutral spirits), malted milk, Ovaltine, Postum and whiskies.

2. *Breads:* Biscuits, crackers, muffins, popovers, pretzels, rolls and the following kinds of breads: corn,*** gluten, graham, pumpernickel, rye, soy and white bread.

   Note: Rye products are not entirely free of wheat. Whether you can use rye will have to be studied as an individual problem, if you are found sensitive to wheat.

3. *Cereals:* Bran flakes, corn flakes, cream of wheat, crackels, farina, Grape-nuts, Krumbles, Muffets, Pep, Pettijohn's puffed wheat, Ralston's wheat cereal, Rice Krispies, Shredded Wheat, Triscuits, Wheatena and other malted cereals.

The inclusion of malted cereals in the wheat list is due to the fact that, for purposes of clinical procedures, barley is considered as being identical with wheat. There are, however, definite sensitizations to barley malt when allergy to wheat cannot be proved. The reverse is also occasionally true.

---

* Permission granted for use by Hollister-Stier Laboratories.
** There are some kinds free of wheat.
** Unless homemade without wheat.

4. *Flours:* Buckwheat flour,* corn flour,* gluten, graham flour, lima bean flour,* patent flour, rice flour,* rye flour, white flour and whole wheat flour. One should not overlook mixtures with flour in them.

5. *Miscellaneous:* Bouillon cubes, chocolate candy and chocolate except bitter cocoa and chocolate, cooked mixed meat dishes, fats used for frying foods rolled in flour, fish rolled in flour, fowl rolled in flour, gravies, griddle cakes, hot cakes, ice cream, malt products or foods containing malt, meat rolled in flour (do not overlook meat fried in frying fat which has been used to fry meats rolled in flour, particularly in restaurants!), most cooked sausages (wieners, bologna, liverwurst, lunch ham, hamburger and so forth), matzos, mayonnaise,* pancake mixtures, sauces, synthetic pepper, some yeasts, thickening creams, waffles, wheat cakes and wheat germ.

6. *Pastries and Desserts:* Cakes, cookies,* doughnuts, frozen pies, pies, chocolate candy, candy bars and puddings.

7. *Wheat Products:* Bread and cracker crumbs, dumplings, hamburger mix, macaroni, noodles, rusk, spaghetti, vermicelli and zwieback.

Important: Prepare foods in separate containers without contacting stuffings, dressings, sauces, gravies, steam-cooking and frying fats. Study the labels of all foods and determine if they contain wheat.

Do not expect the menu in restaurants to be accurate —anticipate this when ordering.

Do not use: Rye, wheatless mixes, "Accent," "Zest" or monosodium glutamate, unless specifically instructed to do so.

---

* Some preparations can be obtained free of wheat.

Eggs*

Egg is found in the following foods and other products:

Baked eggs
Baking powders**
Batters for French frying
Bavarian cream
Boiled dressings
Bouillons
Breads and breaded foods
Cakes
Cake flours
Candies, except hard
Coffee, if cleared with egg
Consommés
Coddled eggs
Cookies**
Creamed eggs
Creamed pies
Croquettes
Custards
Deviled eggs
Dessert powders
Doughnuts
Dried eggs in prepared foods
  and dumplings
Egg albumin
Escalloped eggs
Fried eggs
Fritters
Frostings
French toast
Griddle cakes
Glazed rolls
Hard cooked eggs
Hamburger mix
Hollandaise sauce
Ices
Ice cream
Icings

Laxatives
  Agarol
Macaroons
Malted cocoa drinks (Ovaltine, Cocomalt and others)
Macaroni
Meat Loaf
Meat jellies
Marshmallows
Meat molds
Meringues (French tort)
Noodles**
Omelets
Pastes
Pancakes
Pancake flours
Patties
Poached eggs
Puddings
Pretzels
Salad dressings
Sauces
Sausages
Sherbets
Shirred eggs
Soft cooked eggs
Soufflés
Soups (noodle, mock turtle and consommés)
Spaghetti**
Spanish creams
Tartar sauce
Timbales
Waffles
Waffle mixes
Whips
Wines (many wines are cleared with egg white)

---

* Permission granted for use by Hollister-Stier Laboratories.
** There are some brands free of egg.

You must determine if egg is used in your own brands of pastries, puddings and ice creams. Dried or powdered eggs are often overlooked when inquiry is made!

*Milk**

Milk is found in these foods:

Baking powder biscuits
Baker's bread**
Bavarian cream
Bisques
Blancmange
Boiled salad dressings
Bologna
Butter
Buttermilk
Butter sauces
Cakes
Candies, except hard or homemade
Chocolate or cocoa drinks or mixtures
Chowders
Cookies
Cream
Creamed foods
Cream sauces
Cheeses of every description***
Curd
Custards
Doughnuts
Eggs, scrambled and escalloped

Foods prepared au gratin
Foods fried in butter (fish, poultry, beef and pork)
Flour mixtures, prepared and fritters
Gravies
Hamburgers
Hash
Hard sauces
Hot cakes
Ice creams
Junket
Mashed potatoes
Malted milk
Ovaltine
Ovomalt
Meat loaf
Cooked sausages
Milk chocolate
Milk, including condensed, dried, evaporated, fresh, goat, malted and powdered
Omelets
Oleomargarines
Pie crust made with milk products
Popcorn

---

* Permission granted for use by Hollister-Stier Laboratories.
** Not all preparations contain milk. You must check this. Kosher breads are milk-free.
*** Although all cheeses are to be considered as milk products, a patient not sensitive to milk may be found allergic to one or more cheeses. Therefore, consider each kind and brand of cheese as a potentially specific allergen.

Popovers	Sherbets
Prepared flour mixtures, such as biscuit, cake cookies, doughnuts, muffins, pancakes, pie crust, waffles and puddings	Soda crackers
	Soufflés
	Soups
	Spanish cream
	Spumoni
Rarebits	Whey
Salad dressings, boiled	Waffles
	Zwieback

When you inquire concerning the presence of milk in any product, put your question in this way, "Do you use butter, oleomargarine, cream, cheese of any kind, fresh milk, buttermilk, dried milk, powdered milk, condensed milk, evaporated milk or yoghurt in this food?"

Corn*

Sensitivity to corn is the most common cause of food allergy and, in general, is the most difficult food in the diet to avoid.

1. *Mode of Exposure*

Corn may be a cause of allergic symptoms as the result of ingestion, inhalation or contact. The most common inhalant sources are the fumes of popping corn and the steam of boiling corn on the cob. Other exposures of this nature include inhalation of body powders or bath powders; even ironing starched clothes may be the difficulty. Occasionally, corn is a cause of trouble as an inhalant, when all other sources of corn are tolerated. More rarely, contact exposure to starched clothing or shoes containing corn adhesives will result in symptoms in the highly sensitive individual. In general, the ingestion of corn and corn-containing products represents, by far, the greatest corn exposure.

---

* Permission granted for use by Hollister-Stier Laboratories.

2. *Forms of Corn*

In some instances, there is a difference in the effect of exposure to the different forms of corn. Sometimes, one is able to eat unripe corn without having symptoms, although he will have a reaction if he uses any of the ripe forms or products containing ripe corn fractions, such as sugar, starch or oil.

Variations in sensitization to corn, depending on modes of exposure and forms of corn, are relative differences only. Patients who are so fortunate as to be able to tolerate corn in one manner or form and not in another should report this promptly, in order to receive instructions concerning use of the currently compatible form. Otherwise, complete sensitization may be expected to occur.

The various edible forms of unripe and ripe corn are listed herewith, and, in a subsequent listing, all foods containing corn or made of corn will be given.

A. Ripe Forms of Corn

Corn flakes	Corn syrups
Corn flour	Cartose
Corn meal	Glucose
Corn oil (Mazola)	Karo
Cornstarch	Puretose
Kremel	Sweetose
Linit (often used as food)	Grits
Corn sugars	Hominy
Cerelose	Parched corn
Dextrose	Popped corn
Dyno	

B. Unripe Forms of Corn

Fresh corn	Roasting ears
Canned corn	Fritters
Frozen corn	Succotash

3. *Contacts with Corn*

Corn is used or may be used in a great variety of foods. In fact, it is used in more forms and in the preparations of more kinds of foods than any other single edible product. We have included in our listing all foods in which corn may be used. Your attention is called to the fact that not every brand or all kinds of these foods necessarily contain corn, but many of them do contain it. Any food listed here must be considered as containing corn until a specific individual check indicates that certain brands or types of these foods do not contain corn. You cannot accept the words of untrained persons concerning the presence or absence of corn without specifying by name each of the kinds of ripe corn that may be used. For instance, you must ascertain the following information.

First, ask if any corn sugar, corn syrup or cornstarch is used in the brand of ice cream you wish to use. Ask concerning each of these items by their specific names as given in the list of ripe corn products.

Second, ask if there are any corn sugars or syrups used in your baker's breads and pastries.

Third, ask if corn meal is used in the baking of panless loaves of bread. Corn meal, oatmeal or buckwheat, one or the other, is spread over the hearth before the roll is laid out to be baked. This contact with corn can be eliminated by cutting off the bottom quarter inch of the crust. Do not try to scrape it off!

4. *Treatment of Corn Allergy*

The treatment of allergy requires the complete elimination of corn, all maize products and all foods containing any form or amount of corn. This must be done until you are free of all symptoms. Then it should be determined which, if any, of the refined products can be used. It is imperative for you to receive instructions for the use of unripe corn products, if these are tolerated when the ripe ones cause symptoms. Continued usage of forms of corn which produce negligible or subclinical reactions tends to maintain a high degree of sensitivity. This reduces the possibility of your ever being able to eat corn without having symptoms.

5. *Registration of Corn on the Diet Charts*

Unripe corn is listed as a vegetable. All forms of ripe corn, as well as all foods with corn in any form or amount, are to be listed as corn meal. Do not write in such names as popcorn.

6. *Recommended Products Free of Corn*

Baby Foods: canned meats for babies

Baking Powders and Yeasts: dry yeast

Chocolate Bars

Cocoas

Fruits: All fresh fruits, juice and water-packed; pineapple and pineapple juice; orange juice and tomato juice

Meats: All fresh meats, ham and bacon, canned meats, pork and beans

Paper Cups and Plates: cups (for cold drinks only); paper plates

Pharmaceuticals: Vitamin B, Vitamin C, antihistaminics, capsules

Common Drugs: line of drugs

Vegetables: All fresh vegetables

7. *Foods Containing Corn and Other Corn Contacts*

Adhesives	Tapes	Baking mixes—
Envelopes	Ale	such as
Holiday type stickers	Aspirin and other	A. Biscuits
Stamps	tablets	(Bisquick)
Stickers	Bacon	B. Pie crusts
		(Py-O-My)

C. Doughnuts
D. Pancake mixes
  (Aunt
  Jemima's)
Baking powders
Batters for frying
  Meat
  Fish
  Fowl
Beets, Harvard
Beers
Beverages,
  carbonated
Bleached wheat
  flours*
Bourbon and other
  whiskies
Breads and pastries
Cakes
Candy
Candy bars
Commercial candies
Catsups
Carbonated
  beverages
Cheeses
Cheerios
Chili
Chop suey
Coffee, instant
Cookies
Confectioner's sugar
Corn flakes
Corn Soya
Corn Toasties
Cough syrups
Crackels
Cream O Soy
Cream pies
Cream puffs
Cups, paper
Dates, confection
Deep fat frying
  mixtures
Dentifrices

Excepients or
  diluents in
  Capsules
  Lozenges
  Suppositories
  Tablets
  Vitamins
Flour, bleached*
Foods, fried
French dressing
Fritos
Frostings
Fruits
  Frozen
  Canned
Fruit juices
Frying fats
Gelatin capsules
Gelatin dessert
Glucose products
Graham crackers
Grape juice
Gravies
Grits
Gums, chewing
Gin
Hams
  Cured
  Tenderized
Holiday type stickers
Ices
Ice creams
Inhalants
  Bath powders
  Baby powders
  Cooking fumes of
    fresh corn
  Starch
  Starch—while
    ironing starched
    clothing
Talcums
Jams
Jellies
Jell-o

Kix
Kremel
Leavening agents
  Baking powders
  Yeasts
Linit
Liquors
  Beer
  Bourbon
  Ale
  Gin
  Whiskey
Meats
  Bacon
  Bologna
  Cooked with
    gravies
  Ham, cured or
    tenderized
  Lunch ham
  Sausages, cooked
  Wieners
Milk
Monosodium
  glutamate
Mull-Soy
Nabisco
Nescafe
Oleomargarine
Pastries
  Cakes
  Cupcakes
Peanut butters
Peas, canned
Pies, creamed
Plastic food wrap-
  pers (the inner
  surfaces may be
  coated with
  starch)
Popcorn
Post Toasties
Powdered sugar
Preserves

* Some brands only.

Puddings
  Blancmange
  Custards
  Royal pudding
  Sherbet
Paper containers
  Boxes
  Cups
  Plates (these 3
    only when foods
    have a moist
    phase in contact
    with them)
Rice
  Coated
  Krispies
Salt
Salt cellars in
  restaurants
  A&P Four Seasons
  Salt
Salad dressings

Sandwich spreads
Sauces for
  Sundaes
  Meat
  Fish
  Vegetables
Sausages, cooked or
  table-ready
Sherbet
Soups
  Creamed
  Thickened
  Vegetable
Soybean milks
String beans
  Canned
  Frozen
Sugar, powdered
Syrups, commer-
  cially prepared
  Cartose
  Glucose

Karo
Puretose
Sweetose
Talcums
Teas, instant
Toothpaste
  Craig-Martin and
  Bost
Tortillas
Vanillin
Vegetables
  Canned
  Creamed
  Frozen
Vinegar, distilled
Vitamins
Whiskies
Sobee
Similac
Zest

Allergy Aids*

Here are helps on how to turn that restricted diet into
fun at mealtime with lots of variety. No need to feel
left-out just because certain foods are forbidden. These
recipes can be shared with the whole family. The secret
is in selecting the right foods.

If the allergy is due to wheat or eggs or milk, the
three most common food allergens, food selection may
seem like a major problem, but replacing even these
staple foods can be easy. It just takes a little planning,
and an inquisitive mind when shopping. The stores
are filled with many foods that can be included in
special menus. Browse around and look them over.

Labels on cans and packages usually list the ingredients used. Read the labels carefully. Discover which
foods are wheat-free, corn-free and so forth. For in-

---

* Permission granted for use by General Foods Kitchens.

stance, packaged pudding labels will show if eggs are included and if the thickening agent is cornstarch, wheat, rice flour or tapioca. Syrup labels will indicate the type of sugar the syrup contains, whether cane, corn or maple.

A careful label-reader will soon learn that there are often changes in package contents because of improvements, scarcities and other factors. Read the label of every package before buying.

Sometimes labels may be hard to understand. Words such as "sweetening" and "flavoring" may mean the use of honey, corn syrup or malt flavoring made from various grains. Labeling this way, without listing the individual ingredeints by name, is permitted by the government under the Federal Food, Drugs, and Cosmetic Act.

If additional information is desired on any food labeled in this manner, write to the Food and Drug Administration, U.S. Department of Health, Education and Welfare, Washington, D.C. Request both definitions and standards of identity for the food in question. More information may be obtained from the manufacturer or food-processor. If there is any doubt about a certain food, the doctor should be consulted.

Note to physicians: Information on processing, ingredients and analyses of products made by the General Foods Company is available upon request from General Foods Kitchens, General Foods Corporation, White Plains, N.Y.

Rice, the mainstay in so many allergy meals, can be the most interesting and versatile part of your diet if you use precooked Minute Rice. There is no tedious preparation, and you will have snow-white fluffy rice every time. It is especially delicious when combined with meats and vegetables in savory dishes. Minute Rice picks up the taste and color of the companion ingredients. You will also enjoy Minute Rice with fruit for a milk- egg- and wheat-free dessert.

Fluffy Rice

1⅓ cups (4⅝ ounce package) Minute Rice	½ teaspoon salt
	1⅓ cups boiling water

Add Minute Rice and salt to boiling water in saucepan. Mix just to moisten all rice. Cover and remove from heat. Let stand 5 minutes. Variations: Add 2 tablespoons each of chopped parsley or chives and butter to rice just before serving. Or add ¼ cup of slivered, blanched almonds, sautéed in 2 tablespoons of butter or margarine, or 3 tablespoons of orange marmalade or ¼ cup of chopped, stuffed olives and 2 tablespoons of butter. To make one serving: With Minute Rice it's easy to prepare single servings when needed. Just add ⅓ cup of boiling water to ⅓ cup of rice in a small saucepan. Then mix just to moisten all rice. Cover and remove from heat. Let stand 5 minutes. Makes about ⅔ cup.

Orange Rice

Mix 1⅓ cups of Minute Rice, 1 cup of water, ½ cup of orange juice and 1 teaspoon of salt in a saucepan. Bring quickly to a boil, cover and remove from heat. Let stand 5 minutes. Add 1 teaspoon of grated orange rind, ½ teaspoon of sugar and 2 tablespoons of butter; mix lightly.

Lemon Rice

Prepare 1⅓ cups of Minute Rice as directed on package, adding 1½ teaspoons of grated lemon rind to boiling water with the rice. Just before serving, add

1½ tablespoons of butter; mix lightly. Delicious with broiled or baked fish.

Fruited Rice Pudding

⅔ cup Minute Rice
1¼ cups water
¼ teaspoon salt
¾ cup (about) apricot-applesauce or chopped peaches (or use a 7¾-ounce jar of junior foods)

2½ tablespoons brown sugar
1 tablespoon butter
1 teaspoon lemon juice

Combine all ingredients in saucepan. Cover and simmer 7 minutes, fluffing gently once or twice with a fork. Remove from heat and let stand 5 minutes. Serve warm. Makes 4 servings.

Chicken and Rice

2 tablespoons butter or margarine
½ cup sliced mushrooms, fresh or canned
¼ cup chopped onion
1⅓ cups (4⅝ ounce package) Minute Rice
2 cups chicken broth

1 teaspoon salt
Dash of pepper
1½ cups diced, cooked chicken
¼ teaspoon Worcestershire sauce
½ cup grated cheese (optional)

Melt butter in skillet. Add mushrooms and brown lightly 2 minutes; then add onion and continue cooking until the onion is golden brown. Then add Minute Rice, chicken broth, salt and pepper. Mix just until all rice is moistened. Cover and simmer gently 10 minutes, fluffing rice occasionally with a fork. Add chicken and Worcestershire sauce; heat thoroughly and serve at once, topped with grated cheese. Makes 5 or 6 servings.

Wheat-free? Corn-free? When a substitute is needed for wheat flour or cornstarch, use Minute Tapioca as the thickening agent in stews, cream soups and puddings. And you can make many desserts with Minute Tapioca. Some of them are milk- and egg-free.

Duchess Soup

2 tablespoons minced onion
2 tablespoons butter
2 tablespoons Minute
    Tapioca
1¼ teaspoons salt
⅛ teaspoon pepper

4 cups milk
½ cup grated American
    cheese
2 tablespoons chopped
    parsley

Sauté onion in butter in saucepan until tender. Add
Minute Tapioca, salt, pepper and milk. Cook and stir
over medium heat until mixture comes to a boil. Remove from heat, add cheese and parsley and stir until
cheese is melted. Serves 4 to 6.

Veal Stew

1 pound boned veal shoul-
    der, cut in 1-inch pieces
1 tablespoon fat
2 cups hot water
6 peeled small white onions
4 pared potatoes

1 cup cut green beans
½ cup chopped celery
1½ teaspoons salt
⅛ teaspoon pepper
2½ tablespoons Minute
    Tapioca

Brown veal in fat in heavy saucepan or skillet. Add
water; cover and simmer 30 minutes, or until meat is
almost tender. Add onions, potatoes, beans, celery, salt
and pepper and simmer 30 minutes longer, or until
meat and vegetables are tender. Pour off broth, measure
and add enough water to make 2 cups. Return broth
to meat mixture. Add Minute Tapioca, mix well and
bring to a boil, stirring constantly. Boil briskly 1 minute. Serves 4.

Fluffy Tapioca Cream

Follow directions on Minute Tapioca package to
make fluffy tapioca cream, a luscious dessert whether
served plain or with fruit, nuts, chocolate sauce or
whipped cream. Suggestions for fancy favorites are on
the package.

Fresh Peach Tapioca Pudding

3 tablespoons Minute Tapioca
1/2 cup sugar
1/4 teaspoon salt
1/4 teaspoon nutmeg

1/4 teaspoon cinnamon
3 cups sliced fresh peaches
1 3/4 cups water
1 tablespoon lemon juice
2 tablespoons melted butter

Combine all ingredients, mixing well. Pour into greased 1 1/2-quart baking dish. Bake in moderate oven (375° F.) 40 minutes; stir well every 10 minutes and when removing from oven. Serves 6.

Sunbeam Tapioca

1/4 cup Minute Tapioca
3/4 cup sugar
1/8 teaspoon salt
1/2 cup pineapple juice
1 cup water

1/2 cup orange juice
1 1/2 tablespoons lemon juice
1 orange
1 cup drained, canned pineapple tidbits

Combine Minute Tapioca, sugar, salt, pineapple juice and water in saucepan. Cook and stir over medium heat until mixture comes to a boil. Remove from heat. Add remaining fruit juices. Cool, stirring occasionally. Add fruit, chill. Serves 6.

Variety can be added to your meals with salads and desserts made the Jell-O way. Fruit and vegetable salads, fish molds and Jell-O desserts are all made without wheat, milk and eggs.

Fruited Ruby Flakes

1 package Jell-O (any red
flavor)
1 cup hot water
1 cup cold water

1 banana, sliced
1 orange, sectioned and
diced

Dissolve Jell-O in hot water. Add cold water. Chill until firm. Break into flakes with fork or force through large-meshed sieve. Spoon into a serving dish. Place fruit on top. Serves 4.

Cardinal Pear Mold

1 *package Cherry Jell-O*
1 *cup hot water*
½ *cup cold water*
½ *cup pear juice*

⅛ *teaspoon ginger*
½ *teaspoon salt*
Canned pear halves, cut in thirds

Dissolve Jell-O in hot water. Add cold water, pear juice, ginger and salt. Pour into a mold. Chill until firm. Before serving, unmold and garnish with the sliced pears. Makes 4 servings.

Ginger Ale Salad

1 *package Lemon or Lime Jell-O*
1 *cup hot water*
1 *cup ginger ale*

¼ *cup chopped nuts*
¼ *cup chopped celery*
1 *cup drained, diced, sweetened fresh peaches*

Dissolve Jell-O in hot water. Add ginger ale. Chill until slightly thickened. Then fold in the nuts, celery and peaches. Turn into individual molds. Chill until firm. Unmold on crisp lettuce. Makes 6 servings.

Tuna Fish Salad

1 *package Lemon Jell-O*
1 *cup hot water*
¾ *cup cold water*
1 *tablespoon salad oil*
2 *tablespoons vinegar*
¾ *teaspoon salt*
Dash of pepper
⅛ *teaspoon paprika*

1 *cup (7-ounce can) tuna fish, drained and flaked*
¾ *cup finely diced celery*
2 *tablespoons chopped pimento*
¼ *cup chopped green pepper*
2 *teaspoons prepared horseradish*

Dissolve Jell-O in hot water. Add cold water and chill until slightly thickened. Meanwhile, combine oil, vinegar, salt, pepper and paprika; blend well. Add remaining ingredients and mix thoroughly. Let stand 20 to 30 minutes. Fold fish mixture into slightly thickened Jell-O. Spoon into 8 x 4-inch loaf pan. Chill until firm. Unmold. Cut in slices and serve on crisp lettuce. Makes 6 to 8 servings.

Use Post Toasties to make additional desserts.

Grape Chiffon Pie

3 egg yolks, slightly beaten	3 tablespoons lemon juice
1 cup water	3 egg whites
½ cup sugar	Dash of salt
1 package Grape Jell-O	4 tablespoons sugar
½ cup pineapple juice	1 Toasties pie shell

Mix yolks, water and ½ cup of sugar in saucepan. Cook and stir over low heat until mixture coats metal spoon; cook 1 minute more. (Beat with egg beater if mixture curdles.) Remove from heat. Add Jell-O; stir to dissolve. Add juices; chill until slightly thickened.

Beat egg whites and salt until foamy. Gradually add sugar; beat after each addition. Beat until mixture holds in peaks. Beat Jell-O mixture slightly; fold into meringue; beat slightly. Chill a few minutes until mixture begins to hold shape. Spoon into pie shell. Chill well.

Toasties Pie Shell

Combine 1 cup of finely crushed Post Toasties and 3 tablespoons of sugar in a bowl. Add ⅓ cup of melted butter or margarine; mix well. Press firmly on the bottom and sides of a 9-inch pie pan. Chill 1 hour before filling. Or, if desired, bake pie shell in moderate oven (375° F.) 5 to 8 minutes. Cool before filling.

Toasties Applesauce Dessert

2 tablespoons butter or margarine	3 cups Post Toasties
	2 cups (1 pound) applesauce

Melt butter in skillet. Add Toasties and heat until golden brown, stirring constantly. Place thin layer of

applesauce in shallow serving dish or sherbet glasses.
Add layer of Toasties, then layer of applesauce. Repeat,
topping with layer of Toasties. Serve at once. Serves
4 to 6.

If cocoa and chocolate are off your list but wheat is
all right, try a Postum frosted. Postum is a wheat cereal
beverage and contains no caffein. Or try pull taffy with
Postum.

Postum Frosted

2 tablespoons Instant
    Postum
2 tablespoons sugar

3 cups chilled milk
2 pints vanilla ice cream

Combine all ingredients in bowl, shaker or glass jar
with tight top. Beat thoroughly with an egg beater or
shake well; serve immediately. Makes 4 to 6 servings.

Postum Taffy

2 tablespoons Instant
    Postum
¼ cup boiling water
1 cup white corn syrup

½ cup sugar
⅛ teaspoon salt
1 tablespoon butter or
    margarine

Dissolve Postum in the boiling water. Combine corn
syrup, sugar and salt in saucepan. Add dissolved Postum and place over medium heat until sugar is dissolved,
stirring constantly. Continue cooking without stirring
until a small amount of mixture forms a hard ball in
cold water (or to a temperature of 250° F.). Remove
from heat, add butter and blend well. Pour out on a
buttered platter or shallow pan. Cool until mixture can
be handled. Then pull until light in color and candy
begins to harden. Pull into strip ½ inch thick and cut
with scissors in ½-inch pieces. Makes ¾ pound of taffy.
Store in tightly covered box.

Breakfast

Diets 1 and 2

Approximate Amounts

Beverages:

(a) Grapefruit (fresh) juice or lemonade — 1 *glassful*
(b) Pineapple juice — 1 *glassful*

Cereal:

(a) Boiled brown or polished rice or cooked corn meal served with apricot, peach or prune juice — ½ *cup rice* / 3 *teaspoonfuls juice*
(b) Rice crispies or corn flakes served with grapefruit juice or apricot, peach or prune juice or maple syrup — ¾ *cup dry flakes*
(c) Cold rice or corn meal fried in Mazola oil or bacon or chicken fat, served with maple syrup or Karo corn syrup

Meat:

(a) Bacon (moderately crisp) or — 3 *slices*
(b) Lamb chops, lamb or chicken croquettes (1) ** — 1 *medium chop*
(c) Lamb kidney fried with bacon

Bread:

(a) Corn pone (2) — 2 *muffins or 2 slices toasted*
(b) Corn-rice muffin (3)
(c) Corn-rye muffin (4)
(d) Rice biscuits (5)
(e) Rice bread (6)
(f) Rye bread (7)
(g) Ry-Krisp (8)

*From the writings of Dr. Albert Rowe (with modification)
** Numbers indicate recipes on following pages.

Jams or Preserves:

(a) Peach or prune jam   2 *tablespoon-*
(b) Apricot or apricot-pineapple jam or   *fuls*
    unsweetened preserves
(c) Grapefruit and lemon marmalade
(d) Pear butter (9)

Fruits:

Sliced or whole grapefruit, canned, fresh
    or stewed peaches, apricots, pears,
    pineapple or prunes

Note: Choices as indicated by letters are offered in
all menus though more than one may be used if desired.
Chicken meat and fat should come only from broilers
or roasters. Hens frequently have egg on them as a
result of breaking unlaid eggs in dressing them. Breads,
muffins and cookies should be made at home or by
bakers who follow the recipes given in these diets or
similar ones. Rye flour especially is apt to be mixed
with wheat, and commercial rye bread practically always contains wheat and milk. Corn meal can be
obtained in different degrees of fineness.

This menu contains approximately 922 calories. Also
approximately:

Gm. of carbohydrate	92	Gm. of calcium	0.104
Gm. of protein	16	Gm. of phosphorus	0.200
Gm. of fat	20	Gm. of iron	0.0027

Lunch or Dinner

Diets 1 and 2

Salad:

(a) Lettuce with apricot, pear or pine-   2 *halves or*
    apple with oil dressing or special   *slices*
    mayonnaise

Approximate Amounts

(b) Vegetable salad made of tomato, carrots, beets, asparagus, peas, string beans or artichokes with oil dressing or special mayonnaise
½ cup mixed vegetables
1 tablespoonful oil or dressing

(c) Sliced tomato or lettuce and tomato with oil dressing or special mayonnaise

(d) Lemon gelatin with grated carrots and crushed pineapple

Soup:

(a) Lamb broth clear or with rice, carrot, peas or 1 cup string beans as desired

(b) Chicken broth clear or with rice, carrot, peas or string beans as desired

Meat:

(a) Lamb served as chops, roast or tongue, or stew made with lamb, carrots, peas, beets or string beans
2 medium chops or equivalent

(b) Chicken—roasted, fried, broiled or stewed. May be rubbed with bacon if desired
1 broiler or equivalent

Vegetable:

Spinach, carrots, squash, asparagus, peas, artichokes, beets or tomatoes
4 tablespoonfuls

Bread:

Choice of those in breakfast

Jams or Preserves:

Choice of those in breakfast

Dessert:

(a) Fruit as suggested for breakfast
(b) Rice-fruit pudding (10)
4 tablespoonfuls fruit
(c) Tapioca-fruit pudding (11)
(d) Corn-rice cookies or rice cupcakes (12)
1 cupcake

Approximate Amounts

Beverage:

(a) Grapefruit juice   1 *glassful*
    Corn dextrose may be used if extra
    carbohydrate is desired

Note: It is best to use canned, preserved or freshly
cooked fruits. Uncooked fruits, other than grapefruit
or lemon, are more apt to produce allergic reactions
than heated fruits. Dried fruits well cooked, with the
exception of prunes, are not well tolerated by certain
patients. Soups may be made only with ingredients in
the prescribed diets. Canned soups and those in restaurants and hotels are apt to have wheat, egg or other forbidden ingredients. Meats must not be cooked or based
with any food such as wheat flour, butter or spices not
allowed. Gravies must be thickened only with prescribed flours. Gelatin may be incorporated in salads
and desserts if desired.

This menu contains approximately 864 calories (total
per day—2340 calories). Also, approximately:

Gm. of carbohydrate___125   Gm. of calcium_____0.211
Gm. of protein_____28   Gm. of phosphorus___0.547
Gm. of fat_____28   Gm. of iron_____0.0091

Breakfast

Diet 1

Beverage:

(a) Grapefruit juice   1 *glassful*
(b) Pear juice flavored with lemon   1 *glassful*

Cereal:

(a) Boiled or steamed brown rice served   ½ *cup rice*
    with pear juice or maple syrup   *rice*
                                                  3 *tablespoon-*
                                                    fuls syrup

Approximate Amounts

(b) Rice flakes or rice crispies served with pears or pear — ¾ *cup rice crispies*

4 *tablespoonfuls juice*

(c) Tapioca cooked in water and flavored with lemon juice — 1 *tablespoonful dry tapioca for 1 serving*

Meat:

Lamb chops or patties (13) — 2 *medium chops*

Bread:

(a) Rice biscuits (5) — 2 *biscuits*
(b) Rice bread

Jams or Preserves:

(a) Pear butter (9) — 2 *tablespoonfuls*
(b) Lemon or grapefruit marmalade dietetic

Fruit:

(a) Sectioned or whole grapefruit — 1 *grapefruit*
(b) Fresh or canned pears — 3 *halves*

Note: Corn-sensitive patients often react to corn or gluten which must be excluded even in minute amounts.

This menu contains approximately 768 calories. Also approximately:

Gm. of carbohydrate___118	Gm. of calcium_____0.089
Gm. of protein_____29	Gm. of phosphorus___0.400
Gm. of fat_____20	Gm. of iron_____0.0046

Lunch or Dinner

Diet 1

Salad: Approximate Amounts

  (a) Hearts of lettuce. Dressing of olive   1 *medium head*
      or Wesson oil and Lemon Juice   1 *tablespoon-*
                                     ful oil

  (b) Vegetable salad of lettuce, carrots,   1 *cup mixed*
      beets, artichokes and olives as de-   *vegetables*
      sired with above dressing or special
      mayonnaise

  (c) Lettuce with sectioned grapefruit or   ½ *grapefruit*
      pears served with oil and lemon   *or 2 halves of*
      juice dressing   *pears*

Soup:

Lamb broth clear or with topioca or rice   1 *cupful*
and carrots as desired

Meat:

  (a) Lamb served as chops, roast or ton-   2 *medium lean*
      gue   *chops or*
  (b) Stew made with lamb, rice or carrots   *equivalent*
      or beets

Vegetables:

Steamed or boiled rice, brown   ½ *cup cooked*
Spinach, carrots, beets or artichokes

Bread:

Choice of those suggested for breakfast

Jams or Preserves:

Choice of those suggested for breakfast

Dessert:

  (a) Plain lemon or lime gelatin with
      pears or grapefruit as desired
  (b) Winter pears baked with maple   1 *large pear*
      syrup

Approximate Amounts

(c) Rice cookies or cupcakes (12) (18)   1 *cupcake*
(d) Puffed rice candy (14)
(e) Tapioca-fruit pudding (11)
(f) Rice pudding (10)

Beverage:

Choice of those suggested for breakfast   1 *glassful*

Note: Pure olive oil and Wesson oil only can be used in Diet 1. Imported oil is usually adulterated. Wesson oil and Crisco must be excluded in the presence of positive reactions to cottonseed.

This menu contains approximately 914 calories (total calories per day—2596). Also, approximately:

Gm. of carbohydrate___129   Gm. of calcium_____0.249
Gm. of protein_____32   Gm. of phosphorus___0.557
Gm. of fat_____30   Gm. of iron_____0.010

Breakfast

Diet 2

Beverage:

Approximate Amounts

(a) Pineapple or prune juice   1 *glassful*
(b) Apricot, peach and pineapple juices   1 *glassful*
     mixed
(c) Tomato juice   1 *glassful*

Cereal:

(a) Corn flakes served with pineapple juice or with peaches, apricots or prune juice   4 *tablespoon-fuls juice*
¾ *cup corn flakes*

(b) Corn meal mush served with maple or Karo syrup   ½ *cup cooked cereal*

(c) Cold corn meal mush fried in Mazola oil or bacon fat served with syrup and bacon

Meat: Approximate Amounts

  (a) Bacon   4 *medium strips*
  (b) Chicken croquettes   1 *croquette*

Bread:

  (a) Corn pone (2)
  (b) Corn and rye muffin   2 *muffins*
  (c) Rye bread (7)   1 *or 2 slices*
                                               toasted
  (d) Ry-Krisp (8)   2 *Ry-Krisp*

Jams or Preserves:

  (a) Pineapple preserves   2 *tablespoon-*
                                               fuls
  (b) Apricot or peach jam
  (c) Tomatoes cooked with sugar (15)

Fruit:

Fresh cooked or canned pineapple,   ½ to ¾ *cup*
    peaches, apricots or prunes

This menu contains approximately 856 calories. Also,
approximataely:

Gm. of carbohydrate___149   Gm. of calcium_____0.092
Gm. of protein_____20   Gm of phosphorus___0.279
Gm. of fat_____20   Gm. of iron_____0.0042

Lunch or Dinner

Diet 2

Salad:

  (a) Sliced tomato or asparagus with Ma-   1 *large tomato*
      zola oil and white vinegar or special   *and 6 to 8*
      mayonnaise   *stalks of*
                                                    asparagus

  (b) Combination vegetable salad with   2 *tablespon-*
      tomatoes, asparagus, peas and string   *fuls oil*
      beans as desired, with above oil   1 *cup mixed*
      dressing   *vegetables*

Approximate Amounts

(c) Combination fruit salad of pine-   1 *cup mixed*
apple, peaches and apricots with   *fruits*
special mayonnaise thinned with
pineapple juice

(d) Chicken and pineapple salad mixed
with special mayonnaise (16)

Soup:

(a) Chicken broth clear or with peas,   1 *cupful*
string beans or tomato as desired

(b) Split pea soup (17)

Meat:

(a) Chicken—roasted, fried, broiled or   ½ *broiler or*
stewed. May be brushed with Ma-   *fryer or its*
zola oil and rolled in corn meal if   *equivalent*
desired. Serve broiled peaches, apri-
cots or pineapple with fried or
broiled chicken.

(d) Chicken livers rolled in corn starch
or corn meal and sautéed in Mazola
or Wesson oil

(c) Thick slices of tomato fried or
broiled in oil or bacon fat, served
with strips of bacon

Vegetables:

Tomato, squash, asparagus, peas, string   4 *tablespoon-*
beans or corn   *fuls*

Bread:

Choice of those suggested for breakfast

Jams or Preserves:

Choice of those suggested for breakfast

Dessert:

Approximate Amounts

(a) Fruits as suggested for breakfast — 4 *tablespoonfuls*

(b) Rye cookies (18) — 2 *or 3 cookies*

(c) Fruit-cornstarch pudding with crushed pineapple (19) — 3 *tablespoonfuls*

(d) Jellied prunes with pineapple (20)

This menu contains approximately 1006 calories (total calories per day—2868). Also, approximately:

Gm. of carbohydrate	118	*Gm. of calcium*	0.138
Gm. of protein	30	*Gm. of phosphorus*	0.522
Gm. of fat	46	*Gm. of iron*	0.0092

Breakfast

Diet 3

Beverage:

Approximate Amounts

(a) Grapefruit juice or lemonade with sugar if desired — 1 *glassful*

(b) Tomato juice — 1 *glassful*

Cereal substitutes:

(a) Tapioca cooked with apricot or flavored with lemon, maple sugar (20) — 1 *tablespoonful dry tapioca* / ½ *cupful*

(b) Lima bean flakes served with apricot, peach, prune, or grapefruit juice — ¾ *cup lima bean flakes* / 4 *tablespoonfuls juice*

Meat:

(a) Bacon (moderately crisp) — 4 *slices*

(b) Beefsteak, chipped beef, beef patties or tongue — *Small steak or its equivalent*

Bread:

(a) Lima bean-potato bread (21)   2 *slices toasted*
(b) Lima bean-soybean muffins (22).   2 *muffins*

Jams or Preserves:

(a) Lemon or grapefruit marmalade   2 *tablespoon-*
(b) Peach or apricot jam   *fuls*
(c) Tomato preserves flavored with lemon

Fruit:

(a) Sliced or whole grapefruit   1 *grapefruit*
(b) Fresh, stewed or canned peaches or   4 *tablespoon-*
     apricots   *fuls*
(c) Sliced tomatoes

This menu contains approximately 612 calories. Also, approximately:

Gm. of carbohydrate	149	*Gm. of calcium*	0.130
Gm. of protein	23	*Gm. of phosphorus*	0.500
Gm. of fat	26	*Gm. of iron*	0.0078

Lunch and Dinner

Diet 3

Salad:

(a) Sliced tomato with olive or Wesson   1 *large tomato*
     oil and lemon juice dressing   1 *tablespoonful*
                                              oil

(b) Vegetable salad of carrots, lima   1 *cup vegetables*
     beans, string beans, olives or toma-
     toes as desired with olive or Wesson
     oil dressing or special mayonnaise
     (23)

(c) Fruit salad made of grapefruit,   ½ to ¾ *cup*
     peaches, or apricot with above   *fruit*
     dressings

Soup: Approximate Amounts

(a) Beef bouillon clear or with carrots,   1 *cupful*
     lima beans or tomato

(b) Lima bean soup flavored with bacon
     (24).

Meat:

(a) Beefsteak, roast or tongue   *Average liberal*
                                      serving of meat

(b) Beef stew with potato, carrots, lima
     beans or string beans

(c) Calf or beef liver and bacon

Vegetables:

(a) White or sweet potatoes   1 *medium sized*
                                        potato

(b) Carrots, lima beans, string beans   4 *tablespoon-*
     or tomatoes   *fuls*

Bread:

Choice of those suggested for breakfast

Jams or Preserves:

Choice of those suggested for breakfast

Dessert:

(a) Fruits as suggested for breakfast   4 *tablespoon-*
                                        fuls

(b) Tapioca-fruit pudding (11)

(c) Lima bean-potato flour cookies or   2 *cookies or*
     cupcakes frosted with sugar and   1 *cupcake*
     lemon juice icing (25).

Beverage:

(a) Grapefruit juice or lemonade with   1 *glassful*
     sugar as desired

(b) Tomato juice

This menu contains approximately 901 calories (total calories per day—2724). Also, approximately:

Gm. of carbohydrate	*140*	*Gm. of calcium*	*0.326*
Gm. of protein	*38*	*Gm. of phosphorus*	*0.059*
Gm. of fat	*21*	*Gm. of iron*	*0.0190*

RECIPES

(1)   *Chicken Croquettes*

1 *tablespoon oil or chicken fat*

2 *tablespoons cornstarch*

½ *cup liquid (chicken broth)*

¾ *cup cooked minced chicken*

Salt

Make a sauce of fat, cornstarch and liquid. Add the other ingredients. (Cooked corn meal may be added.) Cool, shape and dip in rye flour or crushed corn flakes. Bake in medium oven or fry in deep fat.

(2)   *Corn Pone*

1 *cup corn meal*

½ *teaspoon salt*

Boiling water

1 *tablespoon Mazola oil*

Carefully pour enough boiling water onto the corn meal to make a stiff mixture, stirring constantly. Add the oil and mix well. Mold into oblong "pones" and fry in hot skillet with enough fat to prevent sticking. When brown on one side, turn and brown on the other side. Serve hot.

(3)   *Corn and Rice Muffins*

⅓ *cup rice flour*

½ *cup yellow corn meal*

2 *tablespoons sugar*

2½ *teaspoons baking powder*

3 *tablespoons Mazola oil*

½ *cup water*

Mix all dry ingredients well, sifting them together four or five times. Add the water and oil. Bake in a hot oven 20 minutes. Makes 6 small muffins.

(4)   *Corn and Rye Muffins*

Use the above recipe but substitute rye flour for rice flour.

(5)   *Rice Biscuits*

Made by the Battle Creek Sanitarium.

(6)   *Rice Bread*

1 *cup rice flour*	1 *tablespoon sugar*
3 *teaspoons baking powder*	½ *teaspoon salt*
2 *tablespoons bacon fat or oil*	¾ *cup water*

Sift all the dry ingredients. Add water and fat. Bake in a loaf pan in a moderate oven.

(7)   *Rye-Rice Bread*

⅓ *cup rye flour*	5 *teaspoons baking powder*
⅔ *cup rice flour*	2 *teaspoons olive oil*
½ *teaspoon salt*	1⅓ *cups water*
6 *teaspoons sugar*	

Sift all the dry ingredients together. Add water and oil. Bake in a loaf pan in a moderate oven for 40 minutes.

(8)   *Ry-Krisp*

Prepared by the Ralston Purina Company.

(9)   *Pear Butter*

Select firm, ripe pears. Peel, core and cut into rather small pieces. To 2 cups of prepared fruit add 1 cup of sugar. Cook slowly, stirring frequently to prevent burning, for 2 hours or until the mixture is quite thick.

(10)   *Rice-Fruit Pudding*

Sauce.

1 *cup sugar*	1¼ *cups boiling water*
2 *tablespoons rice flour*	1 *teaspoon lemon juice or vanilla*
½ *teaspoon salt*	

Mix sugar, salt and cornstarch. Add water and cook until thick. Remove from stove and add flavoring. Add boiled rice and apricots or sliced peaches and serve warm. Reserve some sauce to pour over the pudding.

(11) *Tapioca-Fruit Pudding*

2 *halves peaches, sliced*	2 *teaspoons sugar*
1 *tablespoon dry tapioca*	½ *cup peach juice and water*

Drain peaches and sprinkle with 1 teaspoon of sugar. Cook tapioca in juice and water until it is clear. Add remaining sugar and salt. Line a baking dish with peaches. Fill with tapioca and bake in a moderate oven 20 minutes.

(12) *Rice Cupcakes*

⅔ *cup hot water*	¼ *teaspoon salt*
1½ *cups rice flour*	3 *level tablespoons baking powder*
2 *level tablespoons shortening*	1 *teaspoon vanilla*
¼ *cup sugar*	

Pour hot water over half the flour. Cream sugar and shortening and add to the above mixture, beating well. Add the other ingredients, mixing well. Bake in muffin pans about 20 minutes in a fairly hot oven.

(13) *Lamb Patties*

Ground lamb pressed into small patties. Broiled or fried.

(14) *Puffed Rice Candy*

1 *cup sugar*	¼ *teaspoon salt*
⅓ *cup brown sugar*	1 *teaspoon vanilla*
1 *cup water*	*Puffed rice*

Cook sugar and water until syrupy. Add vanilla and salt. Pour in puffed rice, stirring all the time so that the kernels will be evenly coated. Turn mixture into a greased pan and cut in squares. Keeps well in an air-tight container.

(15)   *Tomatoes Cooked with Sugar*

Select firm, ripe tomatoes, remove the skin, cut in slices and drain an hour or more. For each cup of tomatoes add a cup of sugar and boil until thick, stirring often. Sliced lemon may be added to the tomatoes while cooking.

(16)   *Chicken and Pineapple Salad*

Cut cold, boiled chicken into cubes and marinate for two hours in French dressing or oil and white vinegar and salt. Drain well, mix well with about one-third of its volume of diced pineapple and add special mayonnaise, thinned with pineapple juice to taste.

(17)   *Split Pea Soup*

1 cup green split peas	Diced bacon (crisp)
3 cups water	Salt
1 tablespoon bacon fat	

Cook the peas until they form a smooth purée. Just before serving, add salt, bacon fat and crisply fried bacon.

(18)   *Rye or Rice Cookies*

1 cup rye or rice flour	⅓ teaspoon soda
⅓ cup light molasses (or syrup)	1½ teaspoons baking powder
3 tablespoons Wesson oil	1 tablespoon sugar
¼ teaspoon salt	Water to make a stiff dough

Mix dry ingredients. Add syrup, oil and water. Drop on a greased cookie sheet and bake at 325° F. for 15 minutes.

(19)   *Fruit-Cornstarch Pudding*

1½ cups fruit pulp	2 teaspoons sugar
1½ cups water	5 level teaspoons cornstarch

Cook for one-half hour in the top part of a double boiler.

(20) **Tapioca with Apricots**

6 halves apricots, puréed
2 teaspoons sugar
1 tablespoon dry tapioca
½ cup juice and water

Cook the liquid and tapioca in a double boiler until tapioca is clear. Add apricots and blend well. Serve warm with apricot juice.

(21) **Lima Bean-Potato Muffins or Bread**

⅔ cup potato flour
½ cup lima bean flour
3 teaspoons baking powder
¼ teaspoon salt
4 teaspoons sugar
½ cup water
2 tablespoons shortening

Sift dry ingredients together. Melt fat and add to water; then add slowly to dry ingredients. Put in greased muffin tins and bake at 400° F. for 20 minutes. Serve hot. Makes 10 small muffins.

(22) **Lima Bean-Soybean Bread**

Substitute soybean flour for potato flour in recipe for potato-lima bean bread (21).

(23) **Boiled Mayonnaise**

1 teaspoon sugar
½ teaspoon salt
3 level teaspoons starch
Juice 1 large lemon
⅞ cup boiling water
½ cup Mazola oil

Mix sugar, salt, starch and lemon juice. Add water and cook until thick. Remove from stove and slowly add oil, beating vigorously.

(24) **Puree of Lima Bean Soup**

Wash and soak for a few hours 2 cups of dried lima beans. Cook in plenty of water salted to taste. When beans are well done, put through a sieve. Cook small pieces of bacon (crisp). Add enough bacon drippings and crisp, fried bacon to purée to make palatable.

(25) *Lima Bean-Potato Cake and Cookies*

6 tablespoons lima bean flour	2½ teaspoons baking powder
¾ cup potato flour	½ teaspoon vanilla
5 tablespoons shortening	½ teaspoon lemon extract
½ cup water	Few grains salt
⅔ cup sugar	Few drops yellow coloring

Sift dry ingredients, cream fat and sugars and add dry ingredients and water alternately to creamed mixture. Add flavorings and coloring. Put in greased muffin tins and bake in oven at 430° F. for 30 minutes.

Broiled Fruit

Remove skins from ripe fruit (peaches, apricots and so forth). Cut in half and remove stones. Brush well with olive oil and sprinkle with sugar. Cook under a broiler until delicately browned, turning once. Garnish with chopped mint. Serve with broiled chops or chicken.

Eggless Cake

1½ cups sugar	1 cup milk
2 cups flour	2 tablespoons butter
1 teaspoon Royal baking powder	1 teaspoon vanilla

Beat butter and sugar to cream, add milk, flour, salt and baking powder and beat well. Add flavoring. Mix well. Bake in moderate oven 30 minutes.

Eggless Mayonnaise

¼ cup evaporated milk	1 teaspoon sugar
¼ teaspoon granulated gelatin soaked in 1 teaspoon water	1⅛ teaspoons dry mustard
	Few grains cayenne
	1 cup vegetable or olive oil
1 teaspoon salt	1 tablespoon lemon juice
½ teaspoon paprika	1 tablespoon vinegar

Scald milk in top of double boiler. Add gelatin which has been soaked in water 5 minutes and stir until dissolved. Pour into a bowl and chill until icy cold, then add salt, paprika, sugar, mustard and cayenne. Add oil drop-by-drop until mixture thickens a little. Mix lemon juice and vinegar together. Add alternately with the oil, 1 teaspoon at a time, until all are used, beating thoroughly after each addition. Ingredients should be very cold. While mixing, set the bowl in a pan of ice water. Keep in refrigerator until ready to serve. Makes about 2 cups.

Wheat-free Recipes

In the preparation of breads, muffins and cakes, the following pure flours may be obtained as substitutes for wheat:

Potato starch	*Lister's (casein) flour*
Rye flour	*Cornstarch*
Ry-Krisp	*Barley flour*
Pure buckwheat	*Rice flour*

The following wheat substitute recipes have been used by Vaughn and found to be satisfactory:

Rice Waffles

2 cups rice flour	*½ teaspoon salt*
4 tablespoons melted butter	*4 heaping teaspoons baking*
2 cups sweet milk	* powder*
	2 eggs, separated

Fold in stiff whites last. This will serve 4 people.

Rice Muffins

1 cup rice flour	*5 teaspoons melted butter*
4 eggs beaten very lightly	*3 heaping teaspoons baking*
1 pint sweet milk	* powder (added last)*

Bake in a quick oven. This will make 10 muffins.

Oatmeal Cakes

1 egg	*1 cup rolled oats*
½ cup sugar	*⅓ teaspoon salt*
⅔ tablespoon melted butter	*¼ teaspoon vanilla*

Beat egg until light. Add sugar. Stir in remaining ingredients. Drop by teaspoon on a thoroughly greased pan. Spread into shape with a case knife dipped in cold water. Bake in a moderate oven.

Rye Flour Raised Biscuits

1 *potato, mashed*	1 *teaspoon lard*
1 *yeast cake*	3 *level tablespoons salt*
3 *tablespoons sugar*	2½ *pounds rye flour*

Make sponge of potato, yeast and sugar. Let rise one-half hour. Add lard, salt and flour. Knead 5 minutes and let rise 6 hours. Put in pans, let rise again and bake 40 minutes in moderate oven.

Rye Bread

Sponge	*Dough*
9 *ounces water*	9 *ounces water*
9 *ounces rye flour*	25 *ounces rye flour*
½ *ounce compressed yeast*	½ *ounce salt*

Mix sponge and let stand until it breaks (approximately 2½ hours). Mix well and, as soon as dough is light (which will require approximately 30 minutes), make into loaves and place in greased pans. While rising, moisten dough with a little water or milk to prevent crusting. (This should take about 40 minutes.) Bake 1 hour in a moderate oven.

RYE MUFFINS	RICE MUFFINS
1 *egg*	2 *eggs*
2 *cups milk*	2 *cups milk*
1 *teaspoon salt*	1 *teaspoon salt*
1½ *teaspoons baking powder*	2 *teaspoons butter (heaping)*
1 *tablespoon butter*	2 *teaspoons baking powder*
2 *cups rye flour*	3 *cups rice flour*
Mix as ordinary muffins	*Mix as ordinary muffins*

The most satisfactory muffins are prepared with a mixture of rice and rye flours, since the rice flour is rather too dry and the rye too moist.

Gold Cake (Potato Flour)

½ cup butter
Yolks of 6 eggs
1 cup sugar
1 teaspoon vanilla

½ cup sweet milk
½ teaspoon soda
1 teaspoon cream of tartar
1½ cups potato flour

Beat butter and sugar to a cream, add beaten yolks, dissolve soda in milk and add. Stir in flavoring. Add flour sifted with cream of tartar. Bake in a moderate oven until brown.

Oatmeal Cookies

2 cups brown sugar
¼ teaspoon salt
1¾ cups rolled oats

1 teaspoon baking powder
2 eggs
Butter the size of an egg

Cream butter, sugar, oatmeal and baking powder. Mix well. Drop in small portions from spoon into a large baking pan. Bake in moderate oven until brown. Do not put close together.

POTATO AND RYE MUFFINS

2 eggs, well beaten
¼ cup potato flour
1 heaping teaspoon baking
  powder
¾ cup milk
1 cup rye flour
2 tablespoons butter
Cook in muffin pans

RYE CAKES

2 cups rye flour
1½ cups shredded coconut
1 cup milk
1½ cups sugar
2 tablespoons cocoa
1 teaspoon vanilla
Bake in cookie tins

Rye Loaf Bread

4 cups rye flour
¾ cup rice flour
¾ cup any other substitute
  flour
1 cup riced potatoes, solidly
  packed

1 cake yeast (1 ounce)
1 teaspoon sugar
1 tablespoon salt
1 pint lukewarm sweet milk
1 teaspoon caraway seed
  may be added

Pour milk in mixing bowl, add the sugar and yeast (dissolve in ¼ cup of the lukewarm milk). Stir in the rest of the ingredients and knead until smooth and elastic. Let mixture rise in a warm place until double its bulk. Toss on board, form into loaves, place in pans and let rise again until double its bulk. Bake in a rather hot oven 1 hour or longer until well done. Brush top with water.

Buckwheat Bread

A very passable raised bread may be prepared with pure buckwheat flour, using water or, preferably, milk. Baking soda or yeast may be used. The loaf is a bit heavy, and is best sliced thin and warmed to be served as a "Toast Melba."

Potato Flour Muffins

Separate the whites from the yolks of 4 eggs and beat the whites until they are very stiff and dry. Add a pinch of salt and 1 tablespoonful of sugar to the yolks, which have been beaten, and fold this mixture into the whites. Sift ½ cupful of white potato flour and 1 teaspoon of baking powder together and fold into the egg mixture. Finally, add 2 teaspoonfuls of ice water, turn into ungreased muffin pans and bake in a moderate oven (350° F.) for 15 or 20 minutes.

1. Chicago Dietetic Supply House, Inc.
    1750 West Van Buren Street
    Chicago, Illinois 60612
2. *125 Great Recipes for Allergy Diets*
    (made without eggs, milk or wheat)
    Ronald H. Smithies, Ph.D.
    Director, Good Housekeeping Bureau
    955 Eighth Avenue
    New York, New York 10014
3. *Good Recipes to Brighten the Allergy Diet*
    Home Service Department, Best Foods,
    Division Corn Products Co.
    10 East 56th Street
    New York, New York 10022

26 *The Future of Allergy*

ALLERGY is now an established specialty in medicine and is attracting scientists of a high caliber for basic research in this field. The concept of allergy is well established, and good management of the various allergies is being accomplished.

Allergy is in the beginning of a new era; research may present us with a possible cure or better methods of treatment. The Council of the Allergy Foundation of America has selected six broad areas as most worthy of investigation in fundamental research.

1. *Ways in Which Cells of the Body Are Affected by Antigen-Antibody Reactions.* There are many different kinds of antibodies. Some destroy or neutralize the actions of bacteria or toxins in the human system, and, thus, help to combat infection and maintain good health.

In the allergic person, certain antibodies cause sensitivity to a normally harmless substance or substances. If the person comes in contact with the substance to which he is sensitive (the antigen or allergen), a reaction takes place, and the symptoms of allergy appear.

Whatever the antigen, whether it be simply pollen or a complex drug, we know that certain cells of the body of an allergic person become sensitized. How that happens, and why it happens, we do not know.

Some people are sensitive to many things, and others to none at all. Through a study of the tissue cells we may also find out why this is so.

Finally, treatment which will ultimately curb, halt or prevent allergic reactions will depend upon thorough knowledge of the affected cells.

2. *Ways of Preventing Antibody Formation.* The allergic reaction is caused by the meeting of the sensitizing antibody and the antigen for which it is specific. If one or the other were eliminated, no reaction would occur, and there would be no such thing as allergy.

It would be impossible to eliminate the endless number of substances which act as antigens. If it were possible to prevent the sensitizing antibodies from forming at all, allergy could be completely prevented.

Considerable research is necessary in this area.

3. *Histamine Metabolism.* Histamine is a substance usually stored in inactive state in human tissues. When injected into the skin, it produces a hivelike lesion. Upon microscopic and chemical study, this is comparable to an allergic reaction. In allergic reactions, such as asthma, hay fever and urticaria, histamine (or similar substances) may be the agent responsible for the symptoms. In allergic shock, such as allergy to penicillin, it may be released and cause violent reactions, which may be fatal. The exact nature of these reactions is unknown, and extensive study of the metabolism of histamine may shed new light on the whole subject of allergic disease.

4. *Enzymes.* The study of enzymes has become increasingly important in modern medicine. (The 1955 Nobel Prize in Medicine was awarded for work in this field.) Enzymes are organic substances which help complete chemical changes in the body, like digestion. The action of enzymes seems to be either to produce

sensitization or to destroy it. It may even be that a person is sensitive to his own enzymes.

In any event, the relationship between enzymes and allergic reactions is a significant area of investigation.

5. *Autosensitization.* Autosensitization is the sensitivity of an individual to his own tissues. The possibility of allergic senstization to one's own enzymes is only one example.

Another example of autosensitization at work follows. A man suffers damage to the tissue of an eye and degeneration of the eye begins. Then, for no apparent organic reason, his other eye also begins to degenerate. This may be the result of autosensitization. Today, in such instances, the diseased eye is quickly removed before the process can affect the normal eye.

Numerous diseases of the blood, such as the inability of blood-forming organs to produce adequate numbers of white cells, inability to produce proper clotting agents and excessive bleeding into the tissues, are being studied for autosensitive factors. Similarly, certain liver disturbances and kidney conditions have been shown experimentally in animals to develop from sensitization to extracts from the same or other organs.

The ramifications of this area are endless and need investigation.

6. *Collagen Diseases.* These are degenerative diseases of the connective tissues of the body—those tissues which hold nerves, arteries, muscles and all the other cells of the body in place. The collagen diseases include rheumatic fever, rheumatoid arthritis and other diseases less well known but often fatal, such as periarteritis nodosa and lupus erythematosis. Perhaps multiple sclerosis falls into this category. In the whole field of collagen disease, allergy as a factor needs much more investigation.

Future research will lead us to more knowledge of these six areas and help us to solve the unknowns of allergy.

7. Immunity from the allergic standpoint is being studied very intensively and much evidence is being gathered in the studies of the blood and substances called globulins which pertain to the allergies. But there is much more which needs to be learned to make it an effective tool for doctors.

Appendix

Allergens: The Substances That Cause the Allergies

ALLERGENS, the substances which cause allergy, may be classified into four groups: ingestants, injectants, contactants and inhalants.

Ingestants include chiefly foods and drugs. They are absorbed from the stomach and intestines and carried by the blood to the tissues allergic to them.

The injectants enter the blood stream more directly. Injections of tetanus antitoxin containing horse serum are very common. Penicillin, other injected medications and the stings of insects also enter the blood stream.

Contactants give rise to allergic symptoms by direct contact with the skin or mucous membranes.

The inhalants enter the body through the breathing process.

Insect allergens may actually utilize all of the above means of entering the human body to cause a reaction.

Food Allergies

It is startling to realize that about 20 million of 180 million Americans possess pronounced bodily sensitivities, whereas as many as 80 million show minor idiosyncrasies along the same line.

It is not only interesting but significant to note that an observation of 181 sensitivity patients revealed to Dr. C. H. Eyerman that 36 were sensitive to one food, and 145 to more than one food.

Theoretically, any food can cause a body reaction. Unfortunately, the more common foods are the greatest offenders. This is also true of any other substance, as will be noted in the following pages.

Whether you live to eat or eat to live, the cases concerning foods will probably hold a great deal of fascination for you.

Contact Allergies

Slightly more intricate, but no less important or prevalent, is another kind of bodily sensitivity which is highly interesting because it is intriguing. This concerns reactions which result from the physical contact of the body with various irritants.

Although these particular irritants are sometimes in the form of food, they are apt to fall into any or all of the *animal, vegetable* or *mineral* classes. If there were a million contact irritants known to the medical profession, you could be reasonably certain that there would be as many more yet unrecognized.

It is the last point that makes this phase of the subject intriguing. A physician sleuthing for the cause of some bodily difficulty cannot be positive whether his search is for a known or an unknown. For this reason, the list of test items in general use contains only the irritants that have been found to affect the greatest number of people.

When this list is exhausted and all tests show negative results, the physician is on his own. His solution of the case then depends upon his dexterity, attention to detail, thoroughness and ingenuity in ferreting out leading information. Sometimes the cause of the difficulty is obvious, and a quick solution is reached. There are, on the other hand, conditions which chase the physician down every avenue of possibility before a clue is discovered.

Inhaled or Environmental Allergens

The environmental allergens that produce symptoms involving the upper respiratory tract are numerous. The most common of these will be discussed.

House Dust

Allergy to house dust is the most common cause of perennial rhinitis and asthma. There is in house dust a specific substance that is not related to the specific individual materials in the home. People usually feel worse indoors and at night throughout the year and better when outdoors during the summer months. Symptoms are frequently aggravated during fall and winter; cleaning time is always a source of trouble. Inorganic dusts are usually not allergenic and act as nonspecific irritants. The occupational dusts are usually organic in nature and are important sources of inhalant allergy.

Fungi

The fungi act as allergenic agents in the same manner as pollens, house dust and other allergens. There is no growth or reproduction of the fungi in the host. The allergenic molds are nonpathogenic to man and, to a great extent, to plants also. They are plant saprophytes living mostly on dead and injured vegetation. The usual sources of exposure is outdoors rather than indoors, and production of spores is confined mostly to the frost-free period of the year. Although distribution is universal, it is more prevalent in certain areas where conditions are favorable to growth and dissemination.

The terms "mold" and "fungus" are used interchangeably, although "fungus" is actually more inclusive as it applies to other members of the family, such as yeasts, smuts or rusts, which are fungi but not molds. The molds are more frequently responsible for allergic manifestations.

Fungi are irregular plant masses not differentiated into roots, stems and leaves; they lack chlorophyll and depend for food upon organic matter synthesized by other organisms. They may be unicellular or multicellular. Most of the multicellular fungi consist of cells connected end-to-end to form threads, or hyphae, which branch out irregularly to form a network or mycelium. Fungi reproduce by the development of specialized cells called spores or conidia. From these spores the germ tubes develop. Mold identification is based on the wide difference in the reproductive structure of the spores.

There are three forms of biological relationship based upon the source of food: parasites (pathogens) on animal life—these fungi usually cause skin lesions and include *Trichophyton, Monilia, Epidermophyton* and so forth; plant pathogens—these include rusts and smuts and saprophytes—most important from the standpoint of allergy. They thrive on dead or injured vegetation, and their spores are always found in the soil. Fungi are also abundant on plants, foodstuffs and a variety of other substances. They require little nourishment if there is adequate moisture.

The mildew on textiles is generally due to aspergillus or penicillium. It may grow on awnings, tents, draperies and window shades. Upholstered furniture, especially that stuffed with cotton or kapok, may be a source of molds. Raw cotton with a mold growth is of a cheaper grade, and is used in mattresses and upholstery. Certain fungi are used in commercial preparations of foods, drugs and ferments. Many fungi responsible for allergic symptoms may be derived from environmental organic plant or vegetable matter.

The quantity of fungus spores and their antigenicity are most important factors in exposure. The common ones are: (a) *Alternaria*—a common cause of nasal allergy and bronchial asthma which is, as a rule, in greatest abundance and a most important variety; (b) *Hormodendrum*—common, widely distributed, genetically and antigenically related to *Alternaria;* (c) *Helminthosporium*—of particular importance in agricultural areas; (d) *Aspergillus*—widely distributed (but not in large numbers) , more significant as an environmental allergen with no seasonal variations; (e) *Penicillium*—no seasonal variations and counts are low; (f) *Chaetomium and Phoma*—possibly of environmental significance; (g) *Fusarium*—widely distributed (but counts are low) ; encountered more frequently in the South; seasonal factors are suggested; (h) *Mucorales*—rhizopus and mucor occur sporadically in small number with no seasonal or regional trend and (i) smuts and rusts—spores of these appear constantly in significant number on atmospheric slides and may produce bronchial and nasal symptoms.

Tobacco

There are three factors present in tobacco that make it a very significant cause of allergy and other conditions as well. They are 1) pharmacologic, having the effect of a drug on the person; 2) noxious and irritating quality, and 3) allergic cause of an allergy.

It must be understood that it takes from six months to three years to cure tobacco *before* it is subjected to treatment which give tobacco its characteristic aroma. Substances which are added to the tobacco are licorice, glucose, rum, anise, abd coumarin,. The latter contains other ingredients, such as deer's tongue, tonka bean and molasses. In addition humectants (moisture-pro-

ducing substances) like glycerol tri-ethylene glycol, and
diethylene glycol are also added. These substances influence the composition of smoke.

You can readily see how complex it would be for the
individual patient to determine which particular substances are giving him his disease.

In considering all these facts, what side effects does
nicotine have? What side effect does pyridine cause?
In addition there are chemicals like carbon monoxide,
hydrogen sulfide, hydrocyanic acid and arsenic. These
are contained in most tobaccos and are partially absorbed into the body. There are also minute quantities of other substances which may not be sufficient
to be factors. But these complex "tars" in smoking tobacco have been implicated as a probable cause of
many diseases of the lungs and heart.

It is therefore an absolute must for a tobacco-sensi-
tive person to refrain from smoking and to avoid
smoke-filled places as much as possible.

Animal Epidermal Allergens

Danders and feathers are important causes of respiratory allergy. Danders most contacted are chicken,
duck and goose feathers, cat, dog, cow, horse, rabbit,
goat and sheep. Secondary offenders are rat, mouse,
guinea pig, camel, monkey, hog, parrot, canary and
pigeon. The active substance in animal hairs is the
dander and not the keratin-containing hair itself.

Feathers are, next to dust, the most common excitant
among nonpollen inhalant allergens. Chicken, duck
and goose feathers are most commonly used in pillows,
upholstery and mattresses.

Horse dander is an extremely potent allergen, and
only slight contact is required to cause symptoms. This
sensitivity is more common in farmers, equestrians

and those in contact with animals. This allergen can be contacted through horsehair used as stuffing in mattresses and in upholstered furniture, padding of clothing, making gloves, brushes, hats, ropes, fishing lines, violin bows and wigs.

Cat dander is very potent and is an important cause of respiratory allergy. Commercially, cat hair is encountered in furs, in the lining of caps, gloves and slippers and in toy animals. Furs may be made of pelts of other animals of the cat family, such as leopard, panther, wild cat, jaguar and tiger. Patients sensitive to cat dander may also be sensitive to these danders.

Dog dander is usually contacted from the animal as a household pet, but fur coats, collars, robes and Chinese rugs are also made from such members of the dog family as coyotes, jackals or wolves.

Rabbit hair contact made with the animal itself is usually confined to laboratory workers, breeders or butchers. Rabbit hair is used in pillows, bedding and upholstery, and may be found in hairy toy animals. Commercially, rabbit as "coney" or "lapin" is used as a fur.

Goat hair is used in velvets, upholstery, plushes and cushions. Mohair is made from angora goat hair, and is used on many household articles. Goat hair combined with wool is used in clothing manufacturing. Cashmere and alpaca are made from goat hair, as are Oriental rugs.

Sheep wool is most likely to cause sensitivity symptoms as a result of contact with the animal or with raw material in industry. Physical and chemical treatment of wool for use in fabrics usually renders it inert; symptoms rarely occur from this source.

Cow hair is not uncommonly a cause of respiratory allergy among farmers and dairy or slaughterhouse workers. The most important source of cow hair dander, as regards patients, is the padding used under rugs. Ozite is padding made of cow hair and treated with ozone. Cow hair is also used to make brushes, blankets and rugs. Chenille and Chinese rugs contain cow hair.

Human dander may be a cause of respiratory and skin allergy, such as is occasionally seen in barbers, hairdressers and makers of wigs.

Entomogenous Allergy

Allergic reactions to insects and their products are observed by and known to everyone. Allergic or toxic reactions to the bites of such insects as bees, gnats, chiggers, fleas, mosquitoes and bedbugs are not uncommon. Emanations from insects may produce sensitization by inhalation. Those known to do so are the May fly, sand fly (caddis fly), moth, butterfly, flea and range moth. Also included in this group is silk, a secretion of the mulberry silkworm.

Inhalant Cereal and Grain Dusts

The various cereal flours, such as wheat, corn, oats, barley, rice and buckwheat may cause respiratory allergy. By inhalation, they may affect farmers, bakers, housewives, millers, grocers, feed mill workers or poultry feeders. Cereal dusts are common causes of respiratory allergy in grain farmers.

Orris Root

Orris root is a dried powdered rhizome or root obtained from certain species of the iris family. Because of its fine starch granules, its flesh color and its faint violet scent, it has been used as a base for cosmetics. In addition to face powder, it may also be found in bath powders, facial creams, rouges, perfumes, scented soaps, toilet waters, hair tonics, shampoos, lotions, lipsticks and sachets. Cosmetics advertised as "nonallergic" or "hypoallergic" are generally free of orris root.

Pyrethrum

Pyrethrum is obtained from the dried flowers of certain strains of chrysanthemum. It thus contains pollen and, since the plant is related to ragweed, is more apt to cause nasal symptoms in ragweed-sensitive patients. The drug is used as a principal ingredient in a number of insect powders or sprays, such as those used for fleas, bedbugs and roaches.

Derris Root

Derris root is a substance obtained from the root of a genus of tropical shrubs. It is the important constituent of some insecticides and flea powders. It is used as a dusting powder on vegetable crops. The principal ingredient of derris root is rotenone.

Vegetable Gums

Vegetable gums, including karaya gum, acacia gum and gum tragacanth, are of considerable importance in allergic diseases. The symptoms produced are usually respiratory when the gums are inhaled by sensitive persons. Vegetable gums are obtained from the sap of certain gum trees. The gum most widely used is karaya or Indian tragacanth, obtained from a tree grown largely in India. It is used in a number of popular waveset solutions. Vegetable gums are also used to provide bulk weight in commerically prepared foods, such as fruit pies, ice cream and candies. They are also used as fillers in medications, and as the active principle in many laxatives. They are also employed in printing and in making adhesives and cosmetics.

Cottonseed

It is the water-soluble fraction of cottonseed that is
the potent allergen. Inferior grades of cotton contain
pieces of seed and the linters. This material is used for
stuffing of mattresses, pillows and cushions. Cottonseed
is added to grain and made into stock feed for cattle,
poultry and hogs. It is also used in dog food and as a
flour in the baking industry.

Kapok

Kapok is botanically related to cotton. It is obtained from a plant found in the East Indies and South
America. It is used as stuffing material in cushions, mattresses and upholstery. It is used also in life belts and
preservers.

Flaxseed

This is the seed of the flax plant. It is used in cattle
and poultry feed and in some dog foods. It is also used
in some wavesets, hair rinses, shampoos and tonics.

Glue

Glue may be made from animals and fish, and is used
in woodworking, furniture joints and bookbinding; it
is encountered in sandpaper, sizing for fabrics, carpets
and paper.

Jute

This is a fiber obtained from plants that come from
India. It is used to make burlap bags and also for upholstered furniture, rugs, carpets and carpet pads.

Plastics

Plastic has become an important substance because
of its wide use. It frequently affects the workers who

are in close contact with the complex materials which go to make up the final product. Most of the ingredients cause considerable irritation but some cause strong sensitivity. The ingredients of plastics causing allergy may be summarized as follows:

1. *Resins.* These are contained in nail polish and are known as toluene sulfonamide.

2. *Formaldehyde or phenols.* They are strong sensitizers found in the resins.

3. *Catalysts, stabilizers, hardeners.* These are generally primary irritants and are a widespread hazard to the plastics industry. Hexamethylene tetramine, well-known as a sensitizer, is also used in the rubber industry; phenol, formaldehyde are added to make the manufacture of molded products possible.

4. *Plasticizers.* These increase the flexibility of certain substances. Cellulose and vinyl plastics contain nearly 50 per cent plasticizers. The common plasticizers are O-nitrobiphenyl O- and P-toluene sulfonamide, camphor, tricresyl phosphate, and many of the adipate, stearate, aconitate, sebacate and glycolate esters.

5. *Solvents.* Used primarily for by-products of a liquid nature, such as nail polish, hair lacquers, and varnish, solvents cause both irritation of the skin and allergy. A few solvents are ether, acetone, amyl acetate and compounds from aliphatic alcohols and acetates.

6. *Dyes.* Similar to those used in the textile industry, they are not a common cause of allergy.

The products prepared from these chemicals used in plastics are practically endless—much of our home furnishings, adhesive tape, safety glass, nail polish, paints, wristbands, cords, belts, raincoats, in medicine and dentistry, and so many others too numerous to list.

Allergens Responsible for Sensitization in Industry

I. *In the flour-covering industry:*

1. flaxseed dust
2. cottonseed dust
3. cork dust
4. horsehair
5. cattle hair
6. hog hair
7. sheep hair
8. camel hair
9. llama wool
10. Oriental ox hair
11. hemp dust
12. silk
13. furs (rugs)'
14. powdered glue prepared from expressed fish oils
15. jute dust
16. gum acacia
17. binder twine dust
18. many others

II. *In the pharmaceutical industry:**

1. penicillin, aureomycin, terramycin and other antibiotics in powder form
2. aspirin and other salicylates
3. bath powder
4. vitamins (severe offender)'
5. fish oil derivatives
6. horse serum
7. eggs and egg powder used in preparation of vaccines
8. psyllium
9. cascara bark dust
10. gum tragacanth
11. gum karaya
12. gum acacia
13. dusts of various types of seeds processed:
    a. castor bean dust*
    b. vanilla bean dust
    c. cocoa bean dust
    d. palm seed dust
    e. soybean dust
    f. cottonseed dust
    g. corn dust
    h. sesame dust

*NOTE WELL: In addition to the cathartic factor in the oil, castor bean contains a deadly poison called ricin. This material is present in the nonfatty part of the seed. Ricin is destroyed by heat which the allergen in the bean withstands. All forms of testing with crude castor bean extract are advised against. Extreme and severe local reactions occur after tests with crude castor bean extract. In fact, the ulcerative factor remains even if the ricin in the castor bean is destroyed by heat.

III. *In the fur industry and other industries that process animal danders:*

1. every type of fur dander from mink to muskrat
2. sheep wool
3. goat hair
4. Oriental ox hair
5. hog hair
6. cattle hair
7. llama wool
8. yak hair
9. deer hair
10. mule dander
11. ostrich feathers
12. fowl feathers
13. elk hair

IV. *In the feed and seed industries:*

1. wheat grain dust
2. corn grain dust
3. rye grain dust
4. barley grain dust
5. rice grain dust
6. lentil dust
7. oat grain dust
8. soybean dust
9. cottonseed dust
10. flaxseed dust
11. castor bean dust
12. locust bean dust
13. sunflower seed dust
14. pollens of grasses and weeds
15. grain smuts and other fungi
16. grain elevator dust
17. kafir corn grain dust
18. alfalfa dust
19. mill dust
20. dusts that emanate from hundreds of varieties of seeds when they are processed

V. *In industries that process and use insecticides, there are two types of reaction:*

A. allergic-type reaction, usually to:
   1. pyrethrum
   2. rotenone
   3. tobacco dust
   4. derris root
B. toxic-type reaction to:
   1. methoxychlor
   2. DDT
   3. paradichlorobenzene
   4. benzene hexachloride
   5. chlordane
   6. thallium
   7. toxaphene
   8. lethanes
   9. arsenic preparations
   10. fluorides
   11. nicotine
   12. parathion- and malathion-organic phosphates

VI. *In the vegetable oil industries:*

1. coconut fiber dust
2. cottonseed dust
3. soybean dust
4. castor bean dust
5. flaxseed dust
6. coffee bean dust
7. palm seed dust
8. tung seed dust
9. corn seed dust
10. sesame seed dust

VII. *In the food-processing industry:*

1. grain and seed dusts
2. molds
3. all types of pollens
4. barn dust
5. poultry house dust
6. pyrethrum
7. rotenone
8. danders of various animals processed and so forth
9. popcorn chaff
10. yeasts
11. powdered food dusts
12. dust from all varieties of nuts
13. gum karaya

VIII. *In the home-furnishings industry:*

1. goat hair
2. sheep wool
3. llama wool
4. Oriental ox hair
5. horsehair
6. cattle hair
7. hog hair
8. kapok
9. cotton felt
10. mixed feathers
11. sisal dust
12. silk floss
13. milkweed floss
14. molds
15. glues
16. hemp dust
17. cork dust
18. jute dust
19. leather, all varieties
20. soy bean dust
21. corn dust
22. dusts from other seeds which are used in the manufacture of plastics
23. various types of wood dusts, particularly fir, mahogany, pine, teakwood, cocobola wood
24. volatile paints and varnishes—effect can be both chemical and allergenic

Food Allergens

Alfalfa meal	Apple	Avocado
Allspice	Apricot	Bacon
Almond	Arrowroot	Banana
American cheese	Artichoke	Barley
Anchovy	Asparagus	Bass

Bay leaf
Beef
Beet
Blackberry
Black cap
Black-eyed pea
Black pepper
Black walnut
Bran
Brazil nut
Broccoli
Brussels sprouts
Buckwheat
Cabbage
Calves' liver
Cantaloupe
Caraway seed
Carrot
Cascara bark
Cashew nut
Catfish
Cauliflower
Celery
Cherry
Chestnut
Chicory
Chili pepper
Chive
Chocolate
Cinnamon
Citron
Clam
Clove
Cocoa
Coconut
Codfish
Coffee
Corn
Crab
Cranberry
Crappie fish
Cucumber
Curly kale
Currant
Curry powder
Date

Dill
Duck
Egg (whole)
Egg (white)
Egg (yolk)
Eggplant
Elk meat
Endive
English walnut
Evaporated milk
Fig
Filbert
Flounder
Frog legs
Garlic
Gelatin
Ginger
Goose
Gooseberry
Grape
Grapefruit
Green pepper
     (sweet pepper)
Haddock
Halibut
Herring
Honey
Honeydew melon
Hops
Horseradish
Huckleberry
Juniper berry
Kidney bean
Kohlrabi
Lamb
Leek
Lemon
Lentil
Lettuce
Licorice
Lima bean
Limburger cheese
Lime
Lobster
Loganberry
Mackerel

Malt
Milk (cow)
Milk (cow)
    albumin
Milk (cow) casein
Milk (cow) whey
Milk (goat)
Mint
Mushroom
Mustard
Mutton
Navy bean
Nectarine
Nutmeg
Okra
Oat
Olive (green)
Olive (ripe)
Onion
Orange
Oyster (Eastern)
Oyster (Olympia)
Oyster (Willapoint)
Paprika
Parsley
Parsnip
Pea
Peach
Peanut
Pear
Pecan
Perch
Persimmon
Pickerel
Pike
Pimento
Pineapple
Pistachio
Plum
Popcorn
Poppyseed
Pork
Potato
Prune
Psyllium seed
Pumpkin

Food Allergens (continued)

Quince
Rabbit
Radish
Raisin
Raspberry
Red pepper
   (cayenne)
Red snapper
Rhubarb
Rice
Roquefort cheese
Rutabaga
Rye
Sage
Sago
Salmon
Sardine
Scallops
Sesame seed
Shad
Shrimp

Smelt
Sole
Soybean
Spinach
Squash (banana)
Squash (hubbard)
Squash (Italian)
Squash (summer)
Squash (yellow)
Strawberry
String bean
Sugar beet
Sugar cane
Sweetbreads
Sweet potato
Swiss chard
Swiss cheese
Tangerine
Tapioca
Tea
Thyme

Tomato
Trout
Tuna fish, fresh
Tuna fish, canned
Turkey
Turmeric
Turnip
Vanilla
Veal
Venison
Watercress
Watermelon
Wax bean
Wheat
Wheat (flour)
Whitefish
Yam
Yeast (bakers')
Yeast (brewers')
Youngberry

Epidermal Allergens

Angora wool
Beaver
Camel hair
Canary feathers
Caracul
Cat hair
Cattle hair
Chamois skin
Chicken feathers
Deer hair
Duck feathers
Ermine
Feather mixture

Fox
Fur mixture
Goat hair
Goose feathers
Guinea pig hair
Hog hair
Horse dander
Human hair
Hung, stone marten
Kolinsky
Leopard
Marmot
Mink

Mohair
Muskrat
Nutria
Opossum
Pony
Rabbit hair
Raccoon
Seal (Alaska)
Seal (Hudson)
Sheep wool
Skunk
Squirrel

Smut, Mold and Fungus Allergens

Achorian sch.
Alternaria
Aspergillus flavus
Aspergillus mixture
Aspergillus nudulans
Aspergillus niger
Aspergillus terreus
Botyritis
Cephalosporium
Cerebriforme
Chaetomium globosum
Cheat smut

Cladosporium
Corn smut
Epidermophyton ing.
Fusarium
Helminthosporium
Johnson grass smut
Microsporon Ianosum
Monilia albicans
Monilia sitophilia
Mucor circinelloides
Oat smut
Phoma
Pullularia

Penicillium digitatum
Penicillium expansum
Penicillium glaucum
Penicillium mixture
Penicillium notatum
Penicillium roseum
Rhizopus
Torula pink
Trichophyton
Wheat smut

Miscellaneous Allergens

Alfalfa hay
Aniline
Carbon paper
Cedar
Chalk
Chicle
Cleansing tissue
Coconut fiber
Cod liver
Cotton
Cottonseed
Excelsior
Fir
Flax
Flaxseed
Glue (animal)

Glue (fish)
Grain mill dust
Hemp
Henna
Horse serum
House dust
Jute
Kapok
Karaya gum
Kleenex
Leather
Lycopodium
Newspaper (plain)
Newspaper (color)
Newspaper (rote)
Newspaper mixture

Nylon
Orris root
Pine (white)
Pine (yellow)
Pyrethrum
Quince seed
Rayon
Rice powder
Silk
Sisal
Smoke (cigar)
Smoke (cigarette)
Smoke (tobacco)
Snuff
Tobacco
Upholstery dust

Bacterial Allergens

Aerobacter
  aerogenes
Bacillus coli
Bacillus Friedlander
Bacillus influenzae
Coryne pseudo-
  diphthericum ·
Diplococcus pneumo-
  niae, types 1, 2,
  3, 4, 5, 7
Eberthella typhi
Micrococcus
  catarrhalis

Micrococcus
  tetragenus
Pneumococcus mixed
Proteus X-19
Pyocyaneus
Salmonella paratyphi
Salmonella
  schottmulleri
Shigella flexner
Shigella para-
  dysenteriae
Shigella shiga

Staphylococcus
  albus
Staphylococcus
  aureus
Streptococcus
  fecalis
Streptococcus
  hemolyticus
Streptococcus
  non-hemolyticus
Streptococcus
  viridans

Insect Allergens

Caddis fly
May fly
Wasp
Hornet
Fleas
Moths
Bees

Bedbug
Housefly
Mushroom fly
Mosquito
Body louse
Mites
Ants

Deer fly
Chiggers
Locusts
Citrus fruit fly
Beetles
Yellow jacket

Chemicals and Drug Allergens

1. Paraphenylene diamine
2. Turpentine
3. Mercury bichloride
4. Pyrethrum
5. Nickel sulfate
6. Formalin
7. Quinine hydrochloride
8. Anesthesin
9. Resorcin
10. Potassium dichromate
11. Ammonium fluoride
12. Copper sulfate
13. Potassium iodide
14. Linseed oil
15. DDT
16. Sodium arsenate
17. Butesin picrate
18. Cobalt chloride
19. Chromium chloride
20. Ferris chloride
21. Silver nitrate

22. Zinc chloride
23. Gold chloride
24. Manganese chloride
25. Pure cobalt
26. Ammoniated mercury
27. Crude coal tar
28. Sulfur
29. Sulfathiazole
30. Benzocaine
31. Isocyanatos (Toluyleve),
    2, 4, diisocyanate
32. Platinum salts
33. Oil of cade
34. Salicylic acid
33. Ichthyol
34. Penicillin
35. Aquaphor
36. Benzoic acid
37. Benzyl benzoate
38. Oil of bergamot
39. Beta naphthol

Chemicals and Drugs Allergens (continued)

40. Boric acid
41. Lanolin
42. Viofoam
43. Burrow's solution
44. Balsam of Peru
45. Petrolatum
46. Naftalan
47. Lequor Carbonis Detergens
48. Aureomycin
49. Crysarobin
50. Intracaine
51. Menthol
52. Neomycin
53. Phenol
54. Pragamtar
55. Phenobarbitol
56. Thephorin

Allergens Which Can Cause Skin Allergies (Domestic Vegetation)

Oleoresin Extracts from Ornamental Flowers

1. Bergamot
2. Blue myrtle
3. Calendula
4. Chrysanthemum
5. Coreopsis
6. Cornflower
7. Cosmos
8. Dahlia
9. Feverfew
10. Four o'clock
11. Gaillardia
12. Geranium
13. Hollyhock
14. Iris
15. Jonquil
16. Larkspur
17. Marigold
18. Petunia
19. Primrose
20. Shasta daisy
21. Snapdragon
22. Stock
23. Tansy
24. Verbena
25. Zinnia

Oleoresin Extracts from Ornamental Shrubs and Vines

1. Amoor River privet
2. Arbor vitae
3. Balsam vine
4. Bird of paradise
5. Clematis vine
6. Cypress vine
7. Devil's ivy
8. English ivy
9. Forsythia
10. Grapevine
11. Honeysuckle
12. Lantana
13. Lilac
14. Mock orange
15. Morning glory
16. Oleander
17. Pyrocantha
18. Queen's wreath
19. Salt cedar
20. Scarlet sage
21. Spirea
22. Trumpet vine
23. Virginia creeper
24. Wisteria
25. Yellow jasmine
26. Croton
27. Aurelia
28. Hibiscus
29. Florida Holly

Oleoresin Extract from Fruits, Vegetables and Farm Products

1. Alfalfa
2. Asparagus
3. Broccoli
4. Carrot
5. Celery
6. Corn
7. Flax
8. Grapefruit
9. Green bean
10. Iris potato
11. Lettuce
12. Mustard
13. Oats
14. Okra
15. Orange
16. Parsnip
17. Radish
18. Salsify
19. Sorghum
20. Soybean
21. Spinach
22. Squash
23. Tomato
24. Turnip
25. Wheat
26. Mango
27. Papaya

(Wild Vegetation)

Oleoresin Extracts from Weeds

1. Yarrow
2. Western water hemp
3. Red-root pigweed
4. Short ragweed
5. Smaller burdock
6. Dog fennel
7. Common wormwood
8. Common milkweed
9. Many-flowered aster
10. American thistle
11. Lamb's quarters
12. False ragweed
13. Sneezeweed
14. Sunflower
15. St. John's wort
16. Burweed marsh elder
17. Evening primrose
18. Wild feverfew
19. Black-eyed susan
20. Russian thistle
21. Horse nettle
22. Goldenrod
23. Dandelion
24. Poison ivy
25. Cocklebur

Oleoresin Extracts from Grasses

1. Quack gress
2. Red top
3. Little bluestem
4. Three-awn grass
5. Sideoats grama
6. Downy brome grass
7. Buffalo grass
8. Grass bur
9. Windmill grass
10. Bermuda grass
11. Orchard grass
12. Alkali grass
13. Barnyard grass
14. Wild rye
15. Stink grass
16. Wlid barley
17. Koeler's grass
18. Sprangletop
19. Witch grass
20. Timothy
21. Kentucky bluegrass
22. Foxtail grass
23. Johnson grass
24. Needle grass
25. Crabgrass

Oleoresin Extracts from Trees

1. American elm
2. Ash
3. Basswood
4. Birch
5. Black walnut
6. Box elder
7. Catalpa
8. Chinaberry
9. Cottonwood
10. Hackberry
11. Hickory
12. Honey locust
13. Maple
14. Mesquite
15. Mulberry
16. Oak
17. Osage orange
18. Persimmon
19. Pine
20. Plum
21. Poplar
22. Red cedar
23. Spruce
24. Sycamore
25. Willow

Note Well

The reader should not regard the lists above as complete, as many, many additional substances could be listed. It would require the assistance of a skilled medical detective in this field to find your special allergy if it is not listed above.

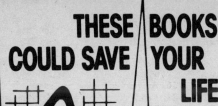
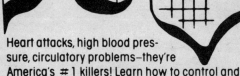